ACSM's Worksite Health Promotion Manual

A Guide to Building and Sustaining Healthy Worksites

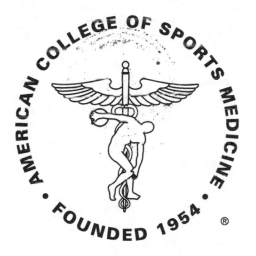

AMERICAN COLLEGE
OF SPORTS MEDICINE

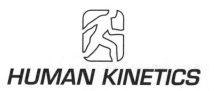

HUMAN KINETICS

Library of Congress Cataloging-in-Publication Data

Cox, Carolyn C., 1960-
    ACSM's worksite health promotion manual : a guide to building and
sustaining healthy worksites / American College of Sports Medicine ;
Carolyn C. Cox.
        p. ; cm.
Includes bibliographical references and index.
    ISBN 0-7360-4657-7 (soft cover)
    1. Employee health promotion--Handbooks, manuals, etc.
    [DNLM: 1. Health Promotion- organization & administration. 2.
Occupational Health. 3. Workplace. WA 400 C8765a 2003] I. Title:
Worksite health promotion manual. II. Title: Guide to building and
sustaining healthy worksites. III. American College of Sports Medicine.
IV. Title
    RC969.H43 C69 2003
    658.3'8--dc21

                    2002013858

ISBN: 0-7360-4657-7

The Web addresses cited in this text were current as of March 2003, unless otherwise noted.

Acquisitions Editor: Scott Wikgren; **Developmental Editor:** Jennifer Clark, **Assistant Editors:** Amanda Gunn and Lee O. Alexander; **Copyeditor:** Ozzievelt Owens; **Proofreader:** Erin Cler; **Indexer:** Patsy Fortney; **Permission Manager:** Dalene Reeder; **Graphic Designer:** Andrew Tietz; **Graphic Artist:** Kathleen Boudreau-Fuoss; **Photo Manager:** Leslie A. Woodrum; **Cover Designer:** Keith Blomberg; **Photographer (interior):** all photographs © Human Kinetics unless otherwise noted; **Art Manager:** Kelly Hendren; **Illustrator:** Accurate Art; **Printer:** Versa Press

Printed in the United States of America   10   9   8   7   6   5   4   3   2   1

Human Kinetics

United States: Human Kinetics
P.O. Box 5076, Champaign, IL 61825-5076
800-747-4457
e-mail: humank@hkusa.com

Canada: Human Kinetics
475 Devonshire Road Unit 100, Windsor, ON N8Y 2L5
800-465-7301 (in Canada only)
e-mail: orders@hkcanada.com

Europe: Human Kinetics
107 Bradford Road, Stanningley, Leeds LS28 6AT, United Kingdom
+44 (0) 113 255 5665
e-mail: hk@hkeurope.com

Australia: Human Kinetics, 57A Price Avenue, Lower Mitcham, South Australia 5062
08 8277 1555
e-mail: liahka@senet.com.au

New Zealand: Human Kinetics
P.O. Box 105-231, Auckland Central
09-523-3462
e-mail: hkp@ihug.co.nz

Visit Human Kinetics on the Web at **www.HumanKinetics.com.**
*For more information about the American College of Sports Medicine and its programs, visit its Web site at **www.acsm.org.***

Contents

Part IV Reengineering for Mature Programs

Part V The Twenty-First-Century Challenge

Contributors

Lisa Bailey
President, Health Promotion Management, Inc.
Broomfield, Colorado

William B. Baun, EPD, FAWHP
The University of Texas M.D. Anderson Cancer Center
Wellness Coach
Houston, Texas

Gary Billotti, MS
Integrated health management leader
Dow Chemical
Health promotion/employee developmental center
Midland, Michigan

Susan Blair, FAWHP
VP business operations
Medifit Corporation
Florham Park, New Jersey

Scott Chovanec
President, Scott Chovanec & Associates
Highland Park, Illinois
Department chair, physical education and health and assistant athletic director
Maine East High School
Park Ridge, Illinois

Carolyn C. Cox, PhD, CHES, FAWHP
Associate professor, health science
Truman State University
Kirksville, Missouri

Tracey L. Cox, FAWHP
Owner
Healing Resources, Inc.
Dallas, Texas

Vicki Diffendal, FAWHP
Manager of health and welfare
Pactiv Corporation
Lake Forest, Illinois

Ron Z. Goetzel, PhD, director
Institute for Health and Productivity Studies
Cornell University
Vice president, consulting and applied research
The MEDSTAT Group
Washington, DC

Thomas Golaszewski, PhD, Associate Professor
SUNY at Brockport
Department of health science
Brockport, New York

John Harris
Principal
Harris HealthTrends, Inc.
Toledo, Ohio

Jacqueline Hooper, DrPH, FAWHP
Dean of health, math, and science
Community College of Denver
Denver, Colorado

David Hunnicutt, PhD
Wellness Councils of America
Omaha, Nebraska

Debbie Jordan
President
Healthy Achievers
Madbury, New Hampshire

Joseph A. Leutzinger, PhD, FAWHP
Union Pacific Railroad
Director, health promotion
Omaha, Nebraska

Susan T. Liebenow
President and co-owner
L&T Health and Fitness
Falls Church, Virginia

Wendy D. Lynch, PhD
Consultant
Lynch Consulting, Ltd
Lakewood, Colorado

Dan Newton
President
The NewSof Group, Inc.
Redmond, Washington

Michael P. O'Donnell, PhD, MBA, MPH
Editor in chief and president
American Journal of Health Promotion
Keego Harbor, Michigan

Ron Ozminkowski, PhD
Director of outcomes and research and econometrics
The MEDSTAT Group
Ann Arbor, Michigan

George Pfeiffer, MS, FAWHP
President
The WorkCare Group, Inc.
Charlottesville, Virginia

Nico Pronk, PhD, FACSM, FAWHP
HealthPartners
Vice President, Center for Health
    Promotion
Research Investigator, Health Partners
    Research Foundation
Minneapolis, Minnesota

Chuck Reynolds
President, employer practice
The Benfield Group
St. Louis, Michigan

Anastasia M. Snelling, PhD, RD, FAWHP
Assistant professor, department of health
    and fitness
American University
Washington, DC

Neal Sofian
CEO
The NewSof Group, Inc.
Seattle, Washington

Maura O. Stevenson, PhD
Associate professor of biology
Community College of Allegheny County
Pittsburgh, Pennsylvania

Paul E. Terry, PhD
Vice president of education
Park Nicollet Institute
St. Louis Park, Minnesota

Gordon R. Waine, FCIB, ACIS
Consultant
Edwalton, Nottingham
The United Kingdom

Ted Wegleitner
Executive director
Park Nicollet HealthSource
Park Nicollet Institute
Minneapolis, Minnesota

Dean Witherspoon
President
Health Enhancement Systems
Midland, Michigan

Preface

Health promotion has often played a secondary role to business and medicine, embraced sincerely and entirely by neither. Medicine tolerates the "wellness" movement as a nice, but not serious, addition to its family of treatments and cures. Businesses alternate between support and rejection of health promotion, depending on current budget requirements and leadership bias. Their complacency stems from the perception that health promotion does not have an immediate relevance to the problems business and medicine face today.

Business and medicine have no trouble supporting the concept of promoting health: Everyone agrees that a healthy lifestyle produces benefits. However, adopting and supporting such activities as a core aspect of the business requires a higher level of commitment from the sponsors. It also requires a widespread and significant level of demand and expectation from consumers. Neither exists. Instead, the focus is the short term. What investments provide a benefit now? What will help me do better today? Health promotion remains ignored because of the belief that the overwhelming majority of consumers won't do what they should do, and for the minority who do, the benefits take time—sometimes years—to achieve.

Relevance defines value. For health promotion, relevance will be critical to future success. How well the field relates its value—to business objectives and medical outcomes, to consumers and corporations, and to everyday performance as well as long-term health—will determine its place in society. Consumer trends in health care–seeking and technology services provide interesting insights about how individuals and companies define value and choose services. Health promotion professionals' ability or inability to establish relevance will define the role of health promotion in the next century.

MAKING HEALTH PROMOTION RELEVANT

Historians remind us of the ways we spent our days 100 years ago. Futurists describe the unimaginable capabilities our grandchildren will experience. Between these past and future visions, we balance the convenience and nuisances created by newly implemented "progress." Pulled by the promise of future scientific advances, we often hold on to beliefs and realities from the past. As a result, sometimes we find ourselves stretched across the gap between what we expect and what we get.

Nowhere are these gaps wider than in our day-to-day interface with health services and with technology. In each area, past delivery systems, even those with historical success and popularity, face a public eager to spend money to find better or faster alternatives. Consumers are turning away from doctors to feel better. Trends indicate quadruple spending for alternative health care and dietary supplements compared with a decade ago. We now spend equivalent (out-of-pocket) sums on alternative and traditional medicine. At a similar pace, consumers are abandoning phone conversations for Internet chats, paper mail for e-mail, and cable for satellite dishes. Experiences with new capabilities and services lead to generalized expectations about how other systems should function. If I can do my banking without waiting for a teller, why can't I get a prescription without waiting for a doctor? If you can put a phone in my home, why can't you provide phone service for my car? If I can take a pill to prevent baldness, why can't I take a pill to prevent obesity? If it costs only $9.99 per month for a satellite to locate my stolen car, why does it cost $1,500 for a doctor to locate my tumor? As consumers, new products redefine our expectations about capability, accessibility, and cost. We expect old systems to keep up.

In a sense, the advances witnessed by the latest generations have produced both a more self-reliant and a more dependent consumer. We can accomplish more with less effort, and—just as easily—find ourselves in trouble. Picture the modern backpacker with a sophisticated global positioning system able to identify his or her position instantly. Picture a patient getting a pacemaker or a transplanted liver functioning independently with diseases he couldn't have survived two generations ago. These miraculous advances provide newfound freedom and opportunity and reinforce a notion that humans can, in many cases, outdo nature. No need to learn about a compass; no need to worry about unhealthy substances such as alcohol or tobacco. Someone will invent a new machine or a cure. Freedom comes with an expectation about safety. The inherent messages are that computers are better than brains, and death is avoidable.

The gap between expectation and reality in health services is partly expectation inflation (a product of media and technology) and partly health service's delay in adopting features of other service industries. Consumers hear daily reports of life-saving and limb-saving advancements, reinforcing the notion of incredible developments in medical science and raising expectations about what medicine can do in extreme situations. For the general public, these expectations easily can be transferred to other aspects of health (e.g., If you can cure something as serious as cancer, certainly you can prevent cavities or colds.). Amazing developments, while eye-catching on the news, rarely apply directly to the consumer and his or her family.

Although shielded somewhat by its effects because of employer contributions for health care coverage, consumers also note reports about the rising cost of health care. Headlines indicate that new advances in procedures and medications cause prices to rise. In efforts to control costs, health plans have placed an increasing number of restrictions on services and prescriptions, making them less accessible to members. In direct contrast to technology, where computers, phones, faxes, and movies-on-demand become even less expensive and more accessible every day, health care heads in the opposite direction. For reasons not well understood by the public, health care remains in continual crisis, medical costs rise, and consumers are asked to settle for fewer and fewer covered services.

Perhaps most important to the expectation gap, health care delivery has virtually ignored the trend of other service industries toward more convenience and better customer service. With few exceptions, health care delivery has maintained a blatant disregard for the time pressures experienced by consumers. Consumers can expect significant delays in service and limited, passive involvement in the treatment options they receive. In no other service area do consumers accept such limitations.

Health care practitioners have, in many cases, reinforced reliance on modern medicine through lowering expectations consumers

should have of themselves. Physicians commonly report a low level of confidence in patients' abilities to manage their own care and a reluctance to trust patients to follow directions. The medical profession reinforces consumer expectations for instant, extrinsic, scientific answers rather than the value of lifelong, simple answers within one's control. The trend toward use of alternative care providers reflects another aspect of the gap between what consumers want and what they get from health care providers. Care seeking involves more than an effort to find the most appropriate treatment solution to a medical issue. Care seeking also includes a search for reassurance and alleviation of discomfort—physical, mental, spiritual, and emotional. Alternative care providers tend to approach discomfort in the more "holistic" sense, incorporating nonphysical aspects of well-being. Consumers seem increasingly more willing to pay for services that are not proved in the context of Western science but provide more healing in the interpersonal sense. By focusing on an overall sense of well-being, alternative providers address more of the underlying causes of care seeking (and health seeking) and increase the relevance and appeal of their services in everyday life.

While consumer expectations about technology or health services may seem disconnected from the business of health promotion, the underlying trends can provide valuable insights and direction for a discipline trying to position itself for the future. Advertisers capitalize on consumer expectations for quick, easy results with promises of weight loss and improved appearance "without the hassles of dieting or exercise." A significant market exists for a variety of unproven electronic devices, pills, and drinks that burn fat without effort. Diet programs attract customers by promising 10 to 15 pounds of weight loss in a single week. It should come as no surprise that sensible lifetime commitments to a regimen of healthy eating and activity have far less appeal. Somehow, health promotion must find a meaningful link with everyday life.

BUILDING THE CASE FOR WORKSITE HEALTH PROMOTION

Many corporations support worksite health promotion, but very few pronounce it as a core business objective. Health promotion does not rise to the top of a corporation's list of business priorities because the short-term value remains invisible. In a business environment where quarterly earnings determine success, few company leaders invest in strategies with a payoff that seems years away. Similar to the purchasing trends of individual consumers trying to improve today's quality of life, employers also have to consider how to improve today's productivity and reduce costs. Again, there are key areas where establishing relevance to the business case may help to position health promotion in the future.

To complete the vision of the health-enhancing workplace, imagine solid evidence that employees who take care of themselves—by eating, exercising, sleeping, and attending to their emotional and spiritual needs in a reasonable fashion—perform better. They think more clearly and creatively, get sick less often, and operate closer to full-work capacity. Imagine evidence that work environments that encourage long hours, skipped meals, and skipped workouts actually reduce overall productivity and retention of talented employees. Imagine social norms that encourage activity and time with family.

Whether these images become reality in the coming decades depends on our ability to establish the relevance of health to how consumers feel and perform *today*. Establishing relevance depends on both the metrics and the

messages health promotion develops in the coming years. Can health-promoting habits provide the feeling of well-being consumers seek (and don't get from traditional care), by either becoming integrated into everyday life, or so enjoyable we make time for them, or by becoming socially or personally relevant and desirable? Can we demonstrate that healthy habits contribute positively to the performance and retention of employees, such that companies value health as an investment in the bottom line?

These questions address some of the crucial challenges and opportunities for worksite health promotion in the future. *ACSM's Worksite Health Promotion Manual* is designed to outline plans, processes, ideas, and examples directly related to the work of building and sustaining these healthy worksites. The text is intended as a resource for all interested or involved in the field of worksite health promotion—from seasoned professionals to college students, from researchers to managed care executives, and from managers to company CEOs. The top experts in the field were brought together to create a resource manual filled with ideas, examples, reflections, experiences, theories, references, and perhaps even some answers that will provide support in formulating program objectives and making sound business decisions that align with the health of companies and the people affiliated with them.

Acknowledgments

Special thanks to the following:

Donald Vickory
Author, physician, and
head of Health Decisions International

Maureen (Mo) Balzer
Wellness and organizational development coordinator
City of Fort Collins, Colorado

Howard Kraft
Manager of benefits education and
health management, Champion

Jan Murnane
Manager of the wellness program
Pitney Bowes

Anita Shaughnessy
Manager of wellness programs
Citibank

Marsha McCabe
Health promotion manager
Texas Instruments

D'Ann Whitehead
Manager, preventive health services
Chevron

Tanya Stott
Star Tribune
Minneapolis, MN
Manager-Worksite Health Promotion

Karyn Entzion
Manager-Worksite Initiatives Center for Health Promotion
HealthPartners

Ann Widtfeldt
Manager-large accounts
Center for Health Promotion
HealthPartners

Michele Adamich
Advisor-Partners for Better Health Initiatives
Center for Health Promotion
HealthPartners

David Bulger
Director
Health Promotion
MicroMass

Introduction

Worksite health promotion is a comprehensive, multidisciplinary, and complex field that seeks to promote, improve, and optimize health, well-being, and performance of those associated with a place of employment. It draws, as a discipline, on a variety of specialized areas such as behavioral and social science, econometrics, organizational learning, business administration, epidemiology, preventive medicine, and political science, to name a few. In all, it brings together the most meaningful set of theories, principles, approaches, and ideas that, as a whole, facilitate the improvement of health.

This task is not easy. It is impossible to be an expert in everything. So, the worksite health promotion professional needs to have a good handle on where to find the information, knowledge, resources, and expertise that are needed to access the underlying foundations on which programs are built, the operational processes that allow programs to flourish, and the motivation to continually keep a heads-up attitude toward new and innovative strategies that allow well-established programs to maintain their cutting edge.

Where do worksite health promotion professionals go for such information? A variety of good information sources exist today in the form of books, newsletters, journal articles, Web sites, and other media. However, a lot of information is presented without a meaningful context. It tends to be fragmented details without a broader application and, often, not based on actual experience in the field. Yet, at the same time, the worksite health promotion field continues to create programs and approaches that are appreciated more and more for their impact on organizational and employee health. In other words, the community of worksite health promotion professionals is creating a very powerful approach to designing, building, implementing, operating, evaluating, researching, and integrating health improvement programs that provide real value for the organizations they serve.

It is the intent of this book to outline theories, models, experiences, and ideas that have originated in the field and present them in a useful manner for the reader. In fact, the reader—yes, that is *you*—is truly the creator of the content presented here. Hence, a manual has been created that presents a set of examples and ideas that reflect on the past (learnings), talk about the present (state of the field), and dream about the future (emerging themes). We have not attempted to present an exhaustive review of all available approaches. Instead, we refer to many of the most common and well-documented examples that exist today, while also taking a peek at what the future may bring.

PURPOSE AND FORMAT OF THE MANUAL

The primary purpose of the *ACSM's Worksite Health Promotion Manual* is to be an easy-to-use practitioner resource that shares theories, models, experiences, ideas, reflections, and anticipated trends related to the

¬ start-up of new programs;

¬ operating processes that allow for effective program management;

¬ methodologies that create long-term success;

¬ motivation and lifelong learning that allows for mature programs to reinvent themselves; and

¬ forces that shape the future of worksite health promotion.

This book is organized around five parts: Part I: Building a Strong Foundation; Part II: Operation Processes That Work; Part III: Development Strategies for Mature Programs; Part IV: Reengineering for Mature Programs; and Part V: The Twenty-First-Century Challenge. Each part consists of several chapters presenting topics that support that section's topic. Each part begins with objectives describing the following:

¬ Purpose. What are the major points to be addressed across all chapters in this section?

¬ Application Points. What are the major points to be made that will allow the information presented in the section to be applied in the field?

¬ Vision. How does the section approach the task of meeting the purpose and what shape will the final product take?

A set of common principles that represent features of worksite health promotion programs that are worthy of note have been identified in each chapter. These common principles provide foundational elements that are applicable to virtually all settings or programs. They also provide an additional set of cross-reference points. Throughout the book, when a principle emerges from the text, an easily recognizable icon representing that principle is printed near it. The icons, the principles, and their definitions are outlined as follows.

INTEGRATION

The incorporation of worksite health promotion goals, objectives, processes, or outcomes as integral parts of other groups or areas within the organization.

PROCESS

An interconnected series of actions, tasks, or steps that progressively lead to a defined endpoint or output. Process improvement initiatives systematically assess where in the series of tasks opportunity exists to enhance the final output.

QUALITY

Quality assessment refers to the determination of the degree of excellence. Quality improvement relates to the process of systematically enhancing the degree of excellence of the final output.

RESOURCES

Resources may come in the form of money, time, people or staff, knowledge, materials, or other sources of supplies or support.

SKILL SETS

Skill refers to the ability to use a learned repertoire of various techniques and abilities to complete specific tasks competently, effectively, and readily at the time they are required or demanded.

We have included integration among the common principles; however, it deserves additional attention. Integration is an important aspect of any program, and as the program matures, integration will complement a program in the way it provides value for other areas of the business. Despite the "feel-good" factor associated with integration, it does not necessarily make the practitioner's task any easier. Once integration occurs, it means that the worksite health promotion staff needs to become increasingly sensitive to annual objectives and accountabilities that relate to other departments or divisions inside the company. If done correctly, the explicit recognition of such dynamic interconnectedness among multiple departments has the capacity to create outstanding departmental or organizational performances. The worksite health promotion staff is uniquely positioned to integrate not only around business objectives but also around its own objectives to value the recognition of and belief in people, to create strong human relationships built on trust and mutual respect, and to bring out the best in the most valuable company assets.

In addition, measurement and evaluation represent important focus areas for those responsible for program success. It is critical to proactively take accountability for program performance. To do so requires ongoing measurement and evaluation activity of various aspects of the program. Process evaluations are necessary to monitor quality and optimize resource use. Measurement of outcomes is needed to show impact and assists in proving the program's worth. Although it may be unrealistic to conduct research studies, the program staff should be familiar with the latest research-related developments in the field, particularly because most research is based on sound theory and proven models. We did not, however, include a chapter on evaluation and measurement. Because evaluation and measurement need to be integral components of all programs, they are addressed in each individual chapter.

Finally, the closer the worksite health promotion program can align itself with the mission and vision of the organization, the more opportunity for long-term success it will have. Such an alignment requires the program to document measurable impacts related to economic performance, health and functional capacity (productivity), and continued broad reach into the population. Without these areas of impact, it will be difficult to show a connection to the revenue generated by the company through product development and sales, thereby reducing the perceived value of the program and jeopardizing the continued allocation of resources. Proving the program's value may involve extending the reach of the program beyond the company walls and pursuing partnerships with community agencies or health plans. Worksite health promotion programs can provide significant value to an organization in many ways. We have to ensure that this value is translated and presented in terms that the key customers of the program's outcomes understand.

Part I

Building a Strong Foundation

Part Objectives

Purpose

- ¬ To provide an overview of the program planning process
- ¬ To describe the formation of internal and external alliances to support planning

Application

- ¬ All interventions and planning should be based on proven theory.
- ¬ Program planning should be conducted by a qualified health promotion professional.
- ¬ Internal and external alliances should be formed to extend limited resources.

Vision

- ¬ Practice based on research and fostering partnerships inside and outside an organization are imperatives for the future.

Chapter 1

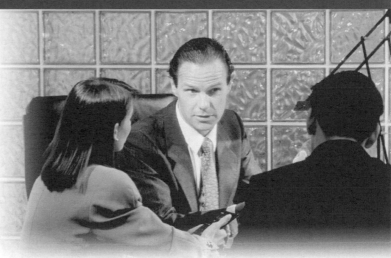

© ICS/Photo Network

Building a Healthy Worksite From the View of a CEO

Many people think of a healthy worksite as one that they themselves do not regard as sufficiently *unhealthy* so as to distract them from their jobs. This definition, in and of itself, is insufficient. Creating a truly *healthy* worksite can have considerable bottom-line business benefits, derived from the motivation, creativity, and general spirit and good health—in its broadest sense—of those who work in the organization. Achieving such a worksite environment is possible but not necessarily easy. It takes time, courage, and the determination of everyone in the organization. Yet the results are worth the effort.

How often does a board of directors or a CEO consider the emotional, mental, and intellectual well-being, in addition to the physical presence, of people in the organization? In today's business environment, it happens way too seldom. When it does happen, the cynic asks, "What does that have to do with business performance?" If there is doubt regarding an individual's absenteeism, the blame is directed toward the employee; blame certainly does not rest on the organization's side.

When the sickness and absenteeism figures are periodically reviewed, there is much the same reaction: "How can we get these figures down? Can we explain this by comparing them to more favorable statistics?" Targeting suspected malingering individuals with thinly veiled threats if they are frequently absent may

be seen as another way of improving numbers or performance.

However, there is a danger of such a vicious circle of hidden agendas, mistrust, blaming others, and indulging personal politics, which contribute to stress and adversely affect business performance.

We can attempt to go beyond simply avoiding an unhealthy worksite and consider creating a healthy one. Health is defined by the World Health Organization (WHO) as ". . . complete physical, mental and social well-being. . . ." We should consider establishing a work environment in which we encourage health from this perspective . . .

WHO's Definition of Health
Health is a state of complete physical, mental, and social well-being and not merely the absence of disease or infirmity (World Health Organization, 1946).

Risking oversimplification, the following model (see figure 1.01) is depicted to illustrate an approach to creating a healthy workplace culture. It includes behaviors, beliefs, attitudes, and values. It is presented as a closed-loop cycle, although the cycle may be entered at any point and is not intended to represent a step-by-step, serially organized set of principles. Rather, the cycle flows according to an intuitive logic that stems from experience and lifelong learning. The model outlines the notion that bringing out the true potential of

3

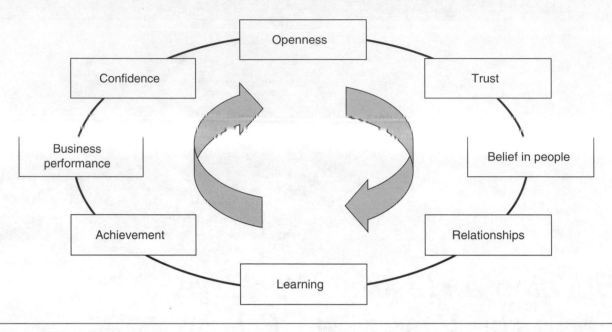

Figure 1.01   Closed-loop cycle.

people within organizations may only be accomplished in an environment that freely incorporates this set of principles in its daily operations.

Considering each component of the model, it is not difficult to see how positive behaviors and outcomes will both benefit the business and lead to higher motivation and personal fulfillment. Furthermore, these results can be achieved in a stimulating, yet demanding, business environment.

Unfortunately, we do not live in an ideal world or work in ideal organizations. Individuals have differing needs and motivations that may get in the way of such a virtuous cycle, and an unhealthy cycle can so easily develop. Personal and business agendas (the latter is often a cover for the former) are often used to take undue advantage of other people, even to the extent of adversely affecting the team as a whole.

Many executives often view this model as a "soft" approach that is likely to give rise to a sloppy and undisciplined attitude among those they see as working *for* them rather than *with* them. They see a need to do things *to* people—to *drive* them and *control* them. If employees do not respond, they are simply "not up to it" or have "their priorities wrong." Such an environment makes it easier to blame others rather than take personal responsibility and show accountability.

Case Study: Richmond Waine; Nottingham, UK

So, what to do? According to Gordon R. Waine, his company Richmond Waine worked the model into the operations of a large banking system over several years by first recognizing that such change is not easy, much less "soft"—it may be a simple approach, but it is certainly not easy. In fact, it turns out to be very difficult work! It takes time, energy, and investment, as well as personal and organizational commitment. Not in the least, it takes courage.

Richmond Waine's executive team followed a set of processes that included the following:

¬ *Surfacing*, or, through a series of conversations, determining what those in the organization—at all levels—see as the most important human and operating values. In other words, what matters most to us in our working lives and to our organization in achieving its mission? To have more than four or five of such values risks diluting what we are trying to achieve. The conversations themselves will ingrain those values that are agreed on among individual employees, who will start to feel that they have a part to play.

¬ *Communicating* the values that have been identified. Who will be affected, both inside the organization and outside the organization? How will they be affected? In what ways can the executive team openly demonstrate its commitment to the process?

¬ *Aligning* the policies and practices of the organization with the agreed on values, beliefs, and attitudes. "Living" this new culture, while providing opportunities for everyone to play a part in creating a healthy workplace, is the really tough part, particularly for a management team with well-established practices and assumptions. Many people may have to change their attitudes and behave differently. Otherwise, cynicism will deepen. Some may be unable or unwilling to change, in which case tough decisions will have to be made. The effectiveness of the process will be severely tested at this stage. The result, however, will be like a breath of fresh air for the organization.

This process is difficult because it allows our own vulnerabilities to show, but it can and does work if the willingness and desire to create a healthy workplace are present, especially in those employees who are ready to emerge as leaders in their areas.

The outcome of implementing this approach is that conversations about complex or sensitive issues become easier. People talk more openly to one another about important organizational, as well as personal, matters. Difficult decisions are readily made rather than avoided in an environment where understanding carries greater force than a fear of reprisal. The quality of personal lives, health of employees (and the sickness and absenteeism figures), and the bottom line all start to improve.

Many details and aspects of such a complex process have not been covered here. We are, after all, talking about an entire system of interacting behaviors, attitudes, values, and beliefs that, taken together, make up a working environment and corporate culture. However, health and business performance are definitely linked. Creating a healthy workplace is fundamental to both. The sense of satisfaction and accomplishment that stems from seeing individuals and their teams fulfilled and personally rewarded through their work while strengthening the health of the organization is immensely rewarding and certainly a CEO's dream come true.

REFERENCE

World Health Organization. 1946. Preamble to the constitution of the WHO as adopted by the International Health Conference, New York. *Official Records of the WHO* 2:100.

Chapter 2

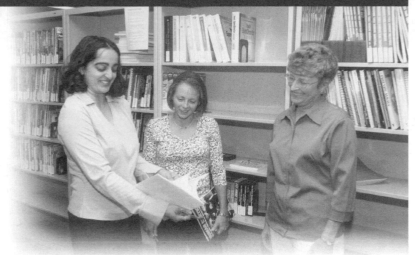

Using Theories and Models to Support Program Planning

Health promotion programs are implemented to improve health and reduce risks associated with disease. Added to the inherent benefits of such programs is an enhancement of the total well-being for individuals, organizations, and communities. Improving individual well-being collectively leads to organizational benefits, such as increased morale, higher productivity, reduced absenteeism, and lower health care costs. For these outcomes to be achieved, however, health promotion programs must be firmly rooted in existing theories and models. These theories and models are best thought of as a systematic method of planning and a decision-making guide.

A theory is a set of interrelated concepts, definitions, and propositions that present a systematic view of events and situations by specifying relations among variables to explain and predict the events or situations (Glanz and Rimer 1997). In other words, theories assist us in understanding (explaining) the health choices individuals make so that health promotion practitioners can more effectively plan programs (predicting).

These efforts, when based on a theory or theories, may aid program development and advancement in the field of health promotion in general. Integral to these theories and models is a flexibility that gives the program planner options or choices to ensure that the program is customized for the organization as the planning process moves forward.

Have you ever asked why, what, and how about programs you have planned? A theory can help explain why people are not coming to a health education program being offered at their workplace. Theories may help determine what elements of a program may appeal to employees. Existing theories guide health promotion practitioners by making us ask critical questions about participants' attitudes and beliefs so that we can later design intervention programs specifically targeted to them. Health promotion practitioners are proactive in a sincere effort to help people change behavior.

As theories are the foundation of the planning process, models are subsets of theories and provide methods by which to apply theories. Effective health promotion programs are based on well-defined models. Models give organization to the program planning process by providing direction as well as structure. Although many different planning models are available, most share common characteristics, albeit with differing viewpoints. Because no one model is perfect, many health promotion practitioners in actual field situations choose to modify or combine aspects of one or more models to create a hybrid model that meets their unique objectives (McKenzie and Smeltzer 1997).

Basic Principles

¬ Theoretical frameworks provide direction for the program and justification for decision making.

¬ Models give structure to the program development process (McKenzie and Smeltzer 1997).

¬ All interventions and program development processes should be grounded in proven theories (McKenzie and Smeltzer 1997) and administered by properly trained health promotion practitioners.

¬ The use of theory helps the health promotion practitioner effectively utilize resources, establish professional credibility (D'Onofrio 1992), and understand motivation and behavior change factors (McKenzie and Smeltzer 1997).

¬ Theories and models are flexible, and they can be modified or expanded to meet specific needs in actual field situations (McKenzie and Smeltzer 1997).

Two general categories of theories and models are directly related to health promotion planning. The first category, behavior change, includes theories and models that help to explain individual and group health behavior. Consideration of these models during planning greatly enhances the development and selection as well as implementation of programs. The second category, program planning, includes theories and models that support the entire program planning process, lending a broader perspective than do those in the behavior change category.

BEHAVIOR CHANGE MODELS

Three theories and models that fall into the behavior change category are the Health Belief model, the Stages of Change theory, and the Social Learning theory. All three are frequently used by health promotion practitioners to enhance their own understanding of the health behavior change process and how to most effectively reach individuals or populations to elicit health behavior change.

HEALTH BELIEF MODEL

The Health Belief model (HBM) was developed in the early 1950s by a group of social psychologists at the United States Public Health Service in an attempt to understand the widespread reluctance of people to access disease prevention services for the early detection of asymptomatic disease (Rosenstock 1974; Janz and Becker 1984). The basic components of the HBM are derived from a well-established body of psychological and behavioral theories whose various models hypothesize that behavior depends on the two following variables:

1. The value placed on a particular goal by an individual.
2. The individual's estimate of the likelihood that a given action will achieve the goal.

The HBM (see table 2.01) includes perceived susceptibility, perceived severity, perceived benefits, perceived barriers, and cues to action.

¬ Perceived susceptibility is a person's perception of the risk of contracting a condition. Individuals vary in their feelings of personal vulnerability to a condition or disease.

¬ Perceived severity is the degree of seriousness of an illness. This component includes the medical consequences of the disease, such as pain, disability, or death, and the social consequences, such as the effect on the family or work.

¬ Perceived benefits involve consideration of whether an identified therapy or program is feasible and efficacious and whether the individual believes he or she can achieve the benefits when action is taken.

¬ Perceived barriers are the potential negative aspects of a particular health action: Is it costly? Is it unpleasant? Is it time-consuming? Is it inconvenient?

¬ Cues to action are the triggers that facilitate the decision-making process. These triggers may be internal or external factors.

STAGES OF CHANGE THEORY

Prochaska, DiClemente, and Norcross proposed the Stages of Change theory

Table 2.01

Application of the Health Belief Model

CONCEPT	DEFINITION	PROGRAM FOCUS
Perceived susceptibility	What is the problem?	Appraise health risk
Perceived severity	What are the consequences?	Identify multiple risk factors
Perceived benefits and barriers	What are the benefits or barriers to taking actions?	Identify opportunities and challenges that support behavior change through discussion
Cues to action	How can the environment support the action?	Alter the environment to support the behavior; provide incentives

after working extensively with smoking cessation and the treatment of drug and alcohol addiction (Prochaska, DiClemente, and Norcross 1992). The basis for the theory is that health behavior is a process and that individuals are at varying levels of readiness for change. Therefore, matching a message with an individual's stage may be more effective for promoting health behavior change than sending out universal messages. Different educational and communication strategies may be used to move people from their current stage to the next appropriate stage. This model (see table 2.02) is considered a spiral model, with people fluctuating through the stages in response to internal and external factors. The stages of change are as follows:

¬ Precontemplation stage. The individual is not thinking about a behavior change.
¬ Contemplation stage. The individual is beginning to recognize the need to change and is considering a behavior change.
¬ Preparation stage. The individual begins to actively seek information about the behavior change process and may experiment with the new behavior.
¬ Action stage. The individual is implementing a plan and is actively changing the behavior.
¬ Maintenance stage. The individual is incorporating the new behavior into his or her lifestyle.

SOCIAL LEARNING THEORY

The Social Learning theory (SLT) was introduced by Miller and Dollard (1941) and later enhanced by Bandura (1986), who renamed it the Social Cognitive theory. Although the SLT is complex, many of its constructs may be useful in the health promotion setting. The underlying premise of the SLT (see table 2.03) is that there is continual interaction between a person and the environment in which the person lives that influences the person's behavior. Consequently, the behavior is dynamic and depends on the interaction between the person and the environment. Therefore, the remaining constructs can be understood by grouping them under personal factors, environmental factors, and behavioral factors.

PROGRAM PLANNING MODELS

The final two models to be reviewed fall into the program planning category. These models provide practitioners with a road map of sorts that directs planning efforts toward successful programs that achieve long-lasting outcomes. The two models that follow are the PRECEDE-PROCEED model and the Social Marketing model.

THE PRECEDE-PROCEED MODEL

The PRECEDE-PROCEED model was designed by Green and Kreuter (1999) for health

Table 2.02

Application of the Stages of Change Theory

CONCEPT	DEFINITION	PROGRAM FOCUS
Precontemplation	Not thinking about physical activity	Raise awareness through lectures and print media
Contemplation	Considering a physical activity program	Assist with how change is made through discussion
Preparation	Investigating a physical activity program	Assist with making specific plans through contracting
Action	Enrolling in a physical activity program	Provide social support and assist with problem solving
Maintenance	Living a physically active life	Assist with preventing relapse

Table 2.03

Application of Social Learning Theory

CONCEPT	DEFINITION	PROGRAM FOCUS
Reciprocal determinism	Continual interaction between the person and the environment	Raise program awareness to individuals and alter the environment to support the behavior
Behavioral capability	Knowledge and skills	Identify knowledge through discussions and print media
Expectations	The value placed on a specific outcome	Highlight the likely results of the behavior
Self-efficacy	Confidence in the ability to take action and accomplish a goal	Identify and support individual strengths
Observational learning	Learning by modeling behavior	Involve leaders in performing the behavior
Reinforcement	Positive or negative triggers for the behavior to be repeated	Provide incentives, rewards, or recognition

promotion programs. This model requires a great deal of analysis before program planning; however, that should not discourage anyone from using it. An understanding of the population, the environment, the health issues, and the available resources is critical, and the model reminds us of the importance of each of these factors when building a strong foundation.

The PRECEDE-PROCEED model has nine phases as described in the following list; the first five phases are diagnostic.

1. Social diagnosis of the self-determined needs, wants, and resources and barriers to them in the target community.
2. Epidemiological diagnosis of the health problems.
3. Behavioral and environmental diagnosis of the specific behaviors and environmental factors for the program to address.
4. Educational and organizational diagnosis of the predisposing, enabling, and reinforcing conditions that immediately affect behavior.
5. Administrative and policy diagnosis of the resources needed and available in the organization, as well as the barriers and supports available in the organization and community.
6. Implementation of the program.
7. Process evaluation of the program.
8. Impact evaluation assesses the immediate results of the program on knowledge, attitudes, and behaviors.
9. Outcome evaluation measures the long-term effects of the program by the change in the quality of life.

SOCIAL MARKETING MODEL

The Social Marketing model was introduced by Kotler and Andreasen (1987) and is based on the commercial marketing practice of focusing on the consumer while the planning, implementing, and evaluating of the program progresses (see table 2.04). Throughout program planning, the importance of a marketing strategy is underscored and continues during the entire process. Central to the Social Marketing model is market segmentation and target marketing. Market segmentation is profiling the audience you are trying to reach, knowing their needs and wants, and understanding their physiological portfolios. Target marketing includes identifying the specific groups you want to reach and positioning the messages to each group.

Target marketing includes knowing the principles of commercial marketing practices by addressing the four "P's" including

¬ price—what the consumer must change to achieve the program benefits;
¬ product—what behavior the program is attempting to change;

¬ promotion—how the message will be communicated; and
¬ place—where the message will reach the target audience.

The major difference between commercial and social marketing is that, rather than selling a product or service, health promotion practitioners are "selling" individual or community behavior change to enhance well-being. However, commercial marketing strategies can be extremely useful in increasing participation and thereby enhancing program effectiveness. The Social Marketing model underscores the importance of the consumer rather than the health issues being the central focus throughout the process. The Social Marketing model allows planners to "sell" health promotion ideas to consumers in such a way that the required commitment of time and effort becomes not only attractive but also desirable.

OVERVIEW OF THE PLANNING PROCESS

The most fundamental steps in the administration of health promotion are planning, implementing, and evaluating. Most writers on the topic emphasize that, although each of these steps involves distinct activities, there is much overlap and all three steps should be ongoing (Simons-Morton, Greene, and Gottlieb 1995). A continuation of planning, implementation, and evaluation results in a highly integrated program that brings about specific health behavior changes that ultimately lead to the desired outcomes.

PRELIMINARY STEPS

Long before specific program decisions are made, several early steps should be followed to gather information that will form a strong foundation for the program. An early review of the evolution of the program using the

---

¬ Who decided that a program should be developed?
¬ What need(s) inspired that decision?
¬ Is the program's champion a single individual, a group, or a company mandate?
¬ What resources, both financial and human, will be made available not only for the implementation of the program but also for the planning and evaluation processes?

Table 2.04

Social Marketing Stages

STAGE	DESCRIPTION
Stage 1: Planning and strategy selection	This stage provides the foundation for the health promotion process, collecting information on health problems, the target audience, goals and objectives, and evaluation measures.
Stage 2: Selecting channels and materials	Planners decide how the target audience will be reached and what materials will be used.
Stage 3: Developing materials and pretesting	Feedback is solicited from the target audience on the materials, messages, and programs developed to address the health problem.
Stage 4: Implementation	The fully developed program is introduced to the target audience.
Stage 5: Assessing effectiveness	The program should be assessed by analyzing the results of measurements.
Stage 6: Feedback to refine program	Information collected throughout the life of the program should be used to refine the program and enhance its effectiveness before it is introduced again.

following questions gives the health promotion practitioner valuable information and insight.

Another decision that should be made early is that of whom to involve in the planning process. It is logical to involve various organizational representatives, but the planning team should not be allowed to grow too large. Otherwise decision making becomes difficult because too many opinions and preferences are involved. That being said, it is wise to consider people from outside as well as inside the organization.

However, it is necessary to ensure that each participant's interest is in improving health among company employees and not in promoting outside products or services. Once the planning partners have been selected, it is a good idea to establish roles and provide assignments (Butler 2001). Having program partners whose areas of expertise are complementary allows for easier division of labor.

Once the planning team has been established and has familiarized themselves with the

factors leading up to the desire for a program, it is time to move into the needs assessment phase. The team will hope to find many "open doors" in this information gathering process. Preliminary courtesy calls can help open these doors, but how does one know whom to contact? It might be a good idea to start with in-house human resources personnel, as well as marketing and facilities personnel. One contact often leads to another. A round of visits can garner support for the planning and eventually for the program. This process also can help the health promotion practitioner feel that he or she is an essential part of the organization in these early phases.

The planning process can take many different forms. However, most approaches focus on a general model for program development that includes the following:

1. Needs assessment
2. Problem identification
3. Goal setting

4. Intervention development
5. Intervention implementation
6. Results evaluation (McKenzie and Smeltzer 1997)

NEEDS ASSESSMENT

Models and manuals provide general guidelines for the planning process, but the most specific and relevant information about the target population will come from a needs assessment. The goal of a needs assessment is to assess the nature of existing problems, concerns, and contributing factors (Simons-Morton et al. 1995). This step allows program planners to analyze the population to be served and to determine the existing health problems of that population.

Failure to conduct a needs assessment can result in the delivery of unneeded educational programs or, worse, the absence of outcomes. Program outcomes that relate to established goals are critical for program survival. The outcomes desired by organizational decision makers must be known and considered as planning moves into the development phase.

A needs assessment can be accomplished in a variety of ways. The complexity of such assessments varies, as does the expense. Regardless of how the assessment is conducted and how much money is spent on it, the data obtained should include demographic information (age, gender, education level, income level, ethnicity, and occupation), incidence of smoking, hospital admissions, causes of death, activity level, infant mortality, and incidence of infectious diseases (Butler 2001).

What are the sources of the needed information? Individual companies may have specific sources such as internal corporate documents. Possible external sources are insurance data, human resource records of other organizations, employee assistance programs, census data, the Centers for Disease Control and Prevention, the National Institutes of Health, and local health organizations (Butler 2001).

In addition to the resources previously mentioned, the program planner may be able to obtain original data via surveys, interviews, and medical examinations and through focus groups. Such methodologies should, of course, adhere to accepted data collection practices such as valid and reliable surveys and interviews, random sampling, and a sample size large enough to allow generalization of findings to the program population (Butler 2001).

Once all the desired data are gathered, organization and analysis are required. Summary statistics can be provided to planning team members before moving on to the next stage, which is the formulation of goals and objectives. A sample of some of the statistics generated after data collection is provided in table 2.05.

Table 2.05

Data Collection–Generated Statistics

POPULATION GENDER	POPULATION AGES	STATISTICS
40% female	Average age = 43.7 yr	60% of the sample population has a cholesterol value that exceeds 200 mg/dl.
60% male	2% < 20 yr 18% = 21–30 yr 30% = 31–40 yr 35% = 41–50 yr 10% = 21–60 yr 4% = 61–70 yr 1% = 71–80 yr	35% of the sample population has a blood pressure reading that is borderline high or higher (140/90).

The data collected during the needs assessment phase are extremely important because they form the basis for the ensuing development not only of goals and objectives but also of programs and materials and of evaluation components as well.

GOALS AND OBJECTIVES

Once needs assessment data are collected and organized, the goals and objectives can be formulated. Known information at this point should be

¬ the population to be served;

¬ the health risks to the population;

¬ education level, occupation, gender, and age of the population;

¬ what kind of health promotion programs the population desires; and

¬ what program outcomes the organizational decision makers desire.

With such information, the planner(s) of the health promotion must ask, "What would we like the program to accomplish?" The broad answer to this question may become the mission statement for the health promotion program (Snelling and Stevenson 1997). More specific answers to this question should pertain to clear and measurable outcomes that will become the program's goals. Goals can be established in a tiered fashion, beginning with broad program goals such as the mission statement and narrowing to specific participant goals. Goals should be further subdivided by specific statements of how the goals will be accomplished; these statements will be the objectives.

The importance of careful attention to this process cannot be overemphasized. Again, the

---

Measurable Goal Example
Goal

Reduce to 30% the number of employees whose cholesterol value exceeds 200 mg/dl.

Objectives

Invite 100% of the individuals whose cholesterol value exceeds 200 mg/dl to attend a cholesterol education series.

Invite 100% of the individuals whose cholesterol value exceeds 200 mg/dl for a follow-up cholesterol test (comparisons can be made between those who attend the course and those who do not).

---

goals and objectives should relate to the needs assessment and certainly should concur with the goals of the sponsoring organization's leadership. The goals must be reasonable and measurable because after a specified period of time (e.g., 6 months or 1 year) progress toward achievement of goals and objectives is measured and documented (see the evaluation section). If necessary, modifications can then be made to program delivery to maintain or improve progress toward goal achievement.

Goals and objectives, once formulated, form the basis for the next step in the planning process: the development and implementation of program offerings and materials.

DEVELOPMENT AND SELECTION OF PROGRAMS

After the initial program planning, the health promotion practitioner will have identified the issues, set the goals and objectives, described the target audience, and identified the available resources allocated for the development and implementation of programs and materials.

Planning the Infrastructure

The first step is to develop the infrastructure to support the program. The primary choices for staffing the program are to hire staff directly as employees of the organization itself (often referred to as in-house staff) or to hire a health promotion contractor for the services. A third alternative would be a combination of these two approaches. Contracting services requires issuance of a request for bids or proposals that invites potential contractors to show how they could manage the program and facility and at what cost. This procedure is frequently seen in government agencies and is often a practical route if the organization has an existing contracts office that is experienced in this type of practice. Hiring staff directly requires a traditional human resources approach that includes development of job descriptions, setting minimum requirements for candidates, establishing salary and other compensation, advertising jobs, and interviewing candidates. In either case, hiring the right staff is a critical element in the long-term success of the program. Staff members should hold a minimum of a bachelor's degree in a health-related field and, depending on the position, have some

14

years of experience in a previous position. A team of professionals with varied backgrounds is ideal.

Another major component of the infrastructure is the facility itself. As one develops facility components such as the exercise area, classrooms, and testing area, one must continually refer to the needs assessment and goals and objectives. Facility components should support the achievement of the goals. If one has the luxury of planning a new facility, the key recommendation is to visit as many other facilities as possible and talk to the professionals who work there.

Development and Selection of Materials

Generally, materials to be developed fall into three primary categories: (1) education, (2) administrative, and (3) evaluation. The programs and materials used to communicate health issues and ultimately motivate individuals toward behavior change should be carefully selected to meet the needs of the audience and achieve the stated goals and objectives. Although programs and materials may appear to offer similar messages, the approaches, graphics, readability, and other factors may have a significantly different impact on behaviors.

Another item that deserves important consideration falls under the category of administrative materials and is known as the informed consent form. This document is to be reviewed and acknowledged via signature by all participants before any involvement in the program. Details of participation should be outlined. For example, if there is a medical screening component to the program, it should be described in detail and any potential risks clearly explained. Details about confidentiality of data should be provided. Participants should know what steps program employees would take to maintain confidentiality. If data are to be used for evaluation purposes, participants should be told how they would be used and reported. Benefits for participation should be noted on the informed consent document along with the statement that participation is voluntary.

PROGRAM IMPLEMENTATION

As programs and materials are developed, individuals who will deliver the programs (e.g., instructors, facilitators, or leaders) should be identified. As resources permit, well-credentialed instructors should be employed and their credentials featured in marketing materials. A number of resources are available to help the health promotion practitioner evaluate potential candidates, and the minimum information obtained from any prospective instructors should include credentials and qualifications, teaching style, and health promotion philosophy.

If time and resources permit, pilot studies of program components should be conducted. Receiving feedback from a small number of pilot participants can be a valuable way to make appropriate changes and "work the bugs out" of intervention before widespread implementation. In the absence of this luxury, an alternative is to phase in program components. This approach involves initially offering the program to only a limited number of people (for example those with the greatest need for an intervention or, in the case of a multisite program, offering the program in a limited number of locations).

This format can offer some of the same benefits as a pilot program and makes implementation more manageable at the start (McKenzie and Smeltzer 1997).

Before the actual commencement of programs, some sort of "kickoff" is a good way to generate enthusiasm. If a facility is being opened, a ribbon cutting ceremony can be held. A program kickoff ceremony can feature a prominent person. Colorful pamphlets, flyers, and posters, as well as slogans can all be used to generate interest.

In-house publications are an excellent method for notifying employees of a program's launch. Newsletters, memoranda, multimedia devices, and notices in employee pay envelopes are also useful.

EVALUATION

It should be noted that health promotion practitioners who have followed the preceding steps have already begun the evaluation process. Scriven (1967) described formative evaluation as the collection and review of data while education programs are still under development. This information helps practitioners form and modify program components before actual implementation.

Too often, evaluation is thought of and dealt with after the fact, when programs are in progress or finishing up. It is critical that the planning of the evaluation process takes place before the fact to ensure that proper data collection takes place. Many new health promotion practitioners have found themselves in the position of starting the evaluation process and realizing too late that the needed objective data are not available.

Although a variety of evaluation categories have been described in the literature, the most widely recognized categories are process, impact, and outcome. Those types will be reviewed here. According to the definitions described by Scriven (1967), these categories would be classified under summative evaluation. This general form of evaluation helps to determine the worthwhile nature of programs after implementation.

Health promotion practitioners as well as the stakeholders need to know what works (Green and Kreuter 1999). As an integral part of the planning process, evaluation can determine program effectiveness or the need for program improvements. Evaluation can answer questions as to whether a program should be modified or continued; can promote improvements during the implementation process; and can assist practitioners in making informed decisions about staff, services, instruction, or activities.

Planning for evaluation begins during the initial program planning, when goals and objectives are being formulated. In addition, the process should be a collaborative effort among stakeholders. To organize the evaluation process, the health promotion practitioner must first include the stakeholders in the process. The scope of the evaluation as well as resource limitations should also be addressed up front. Once the program goals and objectives are formulated, the next steps are to decide which data are to be collected using an appropriate data management system and then to choose a research design. Besides these technical aspects, the health promotion practitioner needs to direct the entire process, interpret the findings to the stakeholders, and use the findings to improve the program (Simons-Morton et al. 1995).

Steps for Selecting the Appropriate Evaluation Design

When planning the evaluation, the health promotion practitioner should use the following steps for selecting the most appropriate research design:

1. Identify program expectations, resources, and constraints.
2. Determine the variables to be evaluated.
3. Decide whether to use a qualitative, quantitative, or combination approach.
4. Choose how to measure the variables; collect, analyze, and report the data (Dignan 1986).

Process Evaluation

For process evaluation, data must be collected to answer questions about intervention content, methods, materials, and instructors. Attendance or participation numbers also fall into the category of process evaluation. Some of the following questions might be answered by conducting a process evaluation:

1. How many participants started the individual programs?
2. How many participants finished the programs?
3. What was the average attendance of the participants?
4. How many participants visited the fitness center for exercise?
5. What was participant satisfaction with the individual instructors?
6. Were materials easy to understand and useful to the education and behavior change process?

Data for process evaluation are obtained through careful record keeping and from questionnaires completed by participants. Computer tracking of data via spreadsheets or databases can make the process infinitely easier than maintaining data by hand. The benefits of process evaluation are many. Results might identify a need to modify the way the program is marketed, the way individuals are targeted, or even simply to change the days or times a class is offered to improve attendance. Results can be used to make decisions about instructors such as whether contracts should be renewed, whether compensation should be increased, or whether content delivery should be modified. Additionally, results from process evaluation may guide the modification of materials in the event that they are difficult to understand or lacking in certain information.

Impact Evaluation

Impact evaluation is performed to determine what if any behavioral and health changes have been elicited from participants in intervention programs. To answer questions about the effectiveness of programs, one must identify changes in participant knowledge, attitude, habits, skills, and motivation. While such information can be very subjective, there are a number of objective measures that should be obtained. For example, some of the information that may be reported after evaluation of the program's impact might be as follows:

1. Average cholesterol before a cholesterol education class compared with after the class (Report the differences in measurement units and as a percentage change.)
2. Blood pressure change
3. Change in health risk (If one uses a health risk appraisal, the change can be calculated.)
4. Number of smokers before a smoking cessation intervention versus after an intervention

As with process evaluation, careful record keeping is critical for successful impact evaluation. Any questionnaires that might be used to collect the more subjective data described must adhere to sound research methodology (i.e., validity and reliability). Preparticipation and postparticipation measurements of particular variables are also important for obtaining objective data for impact evaluation. Clinical measures such as weight, body composition, cholesterol level, and blood pressure are examples of preparticipation and postparticipation measurements that could be considered. However, the variables to be examined should be determined by the stated goals and objectives. For example, if a stated goal was to reduce the number of smokers by a certain percentage, preparticipation and postparticipation evaluations of the number of smokers must be made.

To assess changes in knowledge, attitude, and behavior, it is always preferable to use preparticipation and postparticipation ques-

tionnaires to increase accuracy and reduce bias. The alternative is to ask intervention participants to evaluate changes after completion of a session, but this method lends itself to subjectivity, inaccuracy, and bias. The key to avoiding dependence on such a method is to plan ahead for evaluation and obtain preparticipation measurements.

Results from impact evaluation may be used to guide program planning. For instance, if the evaluation reveals positive changes that are consistent with the stated goals and objectives, the health promotion practitioner may choose to "stay the course" and make minimal changes to the program. However, if goals and objectives are not being met, modifications should be made to get the program on a course that will more likely allow those goals and objectives to be achieved.

Outcome Evaluation

Outcome evaluation moves the health promotion program's effects into a "big picture" perspective and looks at changes that may have occurred in the organization. For outcome evaluation, some terms that may be used are cost-effectiveness, cost benefit, and return on investment. Such an evaluation requires an examination of certain variables in relation to the cost of program implementation. Examples of variables to examine are productivity, absenteeism, employee morale, and utilization of health care. The availability of such information will vary from one organization to the next, but an examination of these factors at the start of the program with a follow-up comparison after 1 year can reveal some improvements that would be of great interest to the decision makers of an organization. Such information may enhance the longevity of their health promotion program or avoid reductions in allocated funds for the program (Snelling and Stevenson 1997). If outcome evaluation is not feasible, one may use existing literature in this area as adjunct support for organization benefits from program outcomes.

Outcome evaluation is often the most challenging form of evaluation for the health promotion practitioner, but careful planning and data collection can make the task not only easier but also much less daunting. A detailing of the steps necessary to accomplish cost-effectiveness or return-on-investment analysis is beyond the scope of this chapter. However, a list of resources available for such evaluation is provided in the bibliography at the end of the chapter.

SUMMARY

In conclusion, successful program development relies on a research base rooted in solid theory. Because of the rapid growth in health promotion research over the past few decades (Wilson 1996; Kaman 1995), health promotion practitioners now have valid theoretical frameworks and models on which to plan their programs. (Simons-Morton et al. 1995).

REFERENCES

Bandura, A. 1986. *Social foundation of thought and action*. Englewood Cliffs, NJ: Prentice Hall.

Butler, J.T. 2001. *Principles of health education and health promotion*. Belmont, CA: Wadsworth Publishing.

Dignan, M. 1986. *Measurement and evaluation of health education*. Springfield, IL: Charles C. Thomas.

D'Onofrio, C.N. 1992. Theory and the empowerment of health education practitioners. *Health Education Quarterly* 19:385-403.

Glanz, K., and B. Rimer. 1997. *Theory at a glance: A guide for health promotion practice*. Washington, DC: U.S. Department of Health and Human Services, National Institutes of Health.

Green, L., and M. Kreuter. 1999. *Health promotion planning: An educational and environmental approach, 3rd edition*. Mountain View, CA: Mayfield.

Janz, N.K., and M. Becker. 1984. The health belief model: A decade later. *Health Education Quarterly* 11:1-47.

Kamam, R.L. (Ed.). 1995. *Worksite health promotion economics: Consensus and analysis*. Champaign, IL: Human Kinetics.

Kotler, P., and A. Andreasen. 1987. *Strategic marketing for nonprofit organizations*. Englewood Cliffs, NJ: Prentice Hall.

McKenzie, J.F., and J.L. Smeltzer. 1997. *Planning, implementing, and evaluating health promotion programs*. Needham Heights, MA: Allyn & Bacon

Miller, N.E., and J. Dollard. 1941. *Social learning and imitation*. New Haven, CT: Yale University Press.

Prochaska, J.O., C.C. DiClemente, and J.C. Norcross. 1992. In search of how people change: Applications to addictive behaviors. *American Psychiatrist* 47:1102-1114.

Rosenstock, I.M. 1974. Historical origins of the health belief model. *Health Education Monographs* 2:2470-2473.

Scriven, M. 1967. The method of evaluation. In *Curriculum evaluation*, ed. R.E. Stake, 160-180. Chicago: Rand McNally.

Simons-Morton, B.G., W. Greene, and N. Gottlieb. 1995. *Introduction to health education and health promotion*. Prospect Heights, IL: Waveland Press.

Snelling, A.M., and M.O. Stevenson. 1997. Writing the annual report: A must for long-lasting programs. *Worksite Health* 4:20-22

Wilson, M.G. 1996. A comprehensive review of the effects of worksite health promotion on health-related outcomes. *American Journal of Health Promotion* 10:429-435.

BIBLIOGRAPHY

Chapman, L. 1996. *Proof positive: An analysis of the cost effectiveness of worksite wellness, 3rd edition*. Seattle, WA: Summex Corporation.

Chenoweth, D. 1998. *Worksite health*. Champaign, IL: Human Kinetics.

Opatz, J. 1994. *Economic impact of worksite health promotion*. Champaign, IL: Human Kinetics.

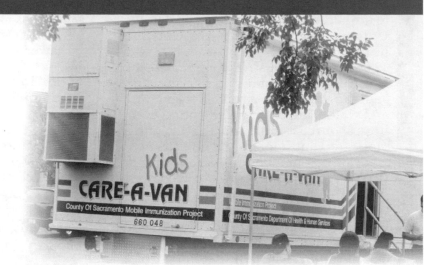

Chapter 3

© Mary Messenger

Forming Alliances to Ensure Program Integration

Once the program is planned, the health promotion practitioner will need to identify internal and external alliances that will facilitate implementation of the plan. These partnerships provide opportunities to cross traditional practice and departmental lines to enhance program visibility, credibility, and accountability, as well as to extend limited resources.

INTERNAL ALLIANCES

Frequently, worksite health promotion programs are designed and implemented in isolation from other departments within a company. Increasingly, worksite health promotion practitioners are becoming aware that to effectively enhance company profitability and worker employability, all programs and policies that are intended to improve organizational and individual health must be integrated with departments such as human resources (personnel, benefits, and training and development), disability management, occupational health and safety, and medical and health services. Collaboration can create unified strategies for meeting the health-related goals of the company.

HUMAN RESOURCES

The names and configurations of services offered by human resource departments differ among organizations. In some organizations, the personnel, benefits, and training and development functions are housed in separate departments, whereas in other organizations, all three units are combined into a single human resource department. Whatever name and configuration a company has for its human resource functions, many cross-functional synergies exist between human resource departments and worksite health promotion.

Keys to making the worksite health promotion and training and development relationship work are as follows:

¬ Keep your eyes open for opportunities for collaboration.

¬ Find out what services are offered by the training and development department, where there are overlaps, and where there are gaps.

¬ Find out what would help the business get where it needs to go.

¬ Expand your knowledge and expertise in stress management.

¬ Develop and expand your expertise and services in other areas. If you can educate and motivate individuals in one area, you can easily do the same in other areas.

Vanderbilt University Case Study

Vanderbilt University believes that the integration of university resources is crucial to the success of HealthPlus, which is the University's comprehensive worksite health promotion program that serves 12,000 faculty and staff. The focus of the HealthPlus program is to assist faculty and staff with improvement in their health and well-being by complementing existing resources and coordinating individual, organizational, and environmental health promotion activities. To ensure the integration of all university resources, the charge to facilitate collaboration between different units was included in the HealthPlus mission statement. In addition to packaging worksite health promotion as an employee benefit that is part of a total compensation package, the University publishes a description of the HealthPlus program and its services in benefit brochures, safety manuals, handbooks, and internal computer listings. Furthermore, the University often includes human resource and health promotion issues in training seminars as well as incorporating health promotion initiatives into events such as the annual football game tailgate celebration (Cavanaugh and Yarborough 1996).

Other nontraditional human resource functions should also be interfaced with worksite health promotion. In particular, because personal financial problems such as home mortgage defaults, bankruptcies, and credit-card delinquency are reaching all-time highs, worksite health promotion programs can offer financial planning in collaboration with the organization's human resource department (Cash 1997). Also, because employee assistance programs specialize in change management, their retirement planning assistance can be coordinated with worksite health promotion programs.

Collaboration Case Study

Are teambuilding, conflict resolution, and organizational development ripe areas for collaboration with worksite health promotion? Absolutely, says Mo Balzer, Wellness and Organizational Development Coordinator for the City of Fort Collins Public Utility located in Colorado. She does not see much difference between a health educator and a trainer except in the content presented. When she first joined the Fort

Collins Public Utility, she developed a 12-session stress management program that covered traditional training topics as well as less traditional stress management topics. To add to her repertoire, she received training in facilitation and mediation skills. Now, instead of just providing a 1-hour presentation for her clientele, including various city departments and managers, she can offer a lead-in presentation, stretch breaks, and facilitation services.

Areas for Collaboration Between Worksite Health Promotion and Human Resources

¬ Benefit plan design

¬ Claims analysis

¬ Liaison with managed care organizations

¬ Training and development

¬ Financial and retirement planning

DISABILITY MANAGEMENT

Another area that has a significant impact on an organization's bottom line is the cost associated with disability. Unscheduled absences caused by a strained back, a complicated pregnancy, or job burnout all affect productivity. When an employee is injured on the job, all worker compensation costs associated with the injury, including the employee's medical costs, lost time, vocational rehabilitation, hiring contractors, and legal action, fall under the disability umbrella. If an employee is not able to perform the essential elements of his or her job, then he or she may be eligible for long-term disability (receiving 50% to 60% of regular pay but not working). All of these examples can take a toll on a company's financial picture.

One large-scale organizational comparison illustrates that the principal determinant of an organization's health and disability experience is its internal management of this area. The quality of management differentiates the best performing organizations from the worst (Barge and Carlson 1993). While external factors such as industry type did explain some of the variability, the most significant finding was that the specific management policies and practices significantly influenced an organization's rate of employee disability, regardless of industry. The characteristics of companies with sig-

Table 3.01

Q Low Versus High Disability Rates

LOW RATE OF DISABILITY	HIGH RATE OF DISABILITY
High employee involvement	Low commitment to safety, health, or disability programs
Positive conflict-resolution strategies	Greater propensity of negative labor-management relations
High organizational commitment to safety, accident prevention, and disability programs and policies	Old school management style and climate
Positive management climate and culture	Low commitment to communication with employees; high employee turnover
Stability in the workforce	

nificantly improved disability and workers' compensation experience compared with companies that had a high rate of costs are listed in table 3.01.

The results of the study demonstrated huge variations in the health and disability costs of the best-managed and worst-managed organizations. Second, there was a wealth of documentation to support the policy of integrated health and disability management strategies. Additionally, with decreasing work stability and increased job demands, it seems unlikely that the strategies used in the past to manage costs will be effective in today's workforce. However, therein lies a huge opportunity to manage these costs. Successful implementation of an integrated disability management process results in a healthier and more productive workforce.

Union Pacific Railroad Case Study

For the past decade, Union Pacific Railroad has implemented successful disability management strategies that affect employees both before an injury takes place and after an employee is injured and is in need of medical attention and vocational rehabilitation (The Health Project, Inc., 2002). These strategies and projects are presented in the following list. "Integrating our health promotion program within our Disability Management Department

has been one of our most successful integration efforts," reports Dr. Joe Leutzinger, who is the Health Promotion Director at Union Pacific Railroad. The results are proof enough:

¬ No new injuries were reported after a 3-year follow-up period for employees who participated in a vocational rehabilitation program who were at risk for injury.

¬ Since 1991, 80% of disabled workers returned to their preinjury job.

¬ Savings of over $16 million in avoided payments and lawsuits was realized.

¬ The number of physicians per case decreased.

¬ The number of lost workdays decreased.

Pitney Bowes Case Study

Using an integrated data system to analyze their short-term disability experience, Pitney Bowes determined that maternity payments per episode were increasing because of the rise in the incidence of complicated maternity cases. As a result, they set out to enhance their maternity management initiatives by combining a prenatal care program with managed disability efforts. Jan Murnane, manager of Pitney Bowes's Wellness Program, indicated that the company contracted with an outside vendor to implement the prenatal program for employees and spouses located in the state of Connecticut. The prenatal program called Great Expectations, managed by the Wellness Program, consists of risk assessments, a 24 hour information line that continues to 6 weeks postpartum, subsidy for breast pumps, discounts on baby products, "health care university credit" discounts on the following year's medical plan, and educational information and support. Results demonstrated that the program was successful in achieving better birth outcomes (e.g., fewer cesarean sections and fewer occurrences of premature deliveries and low-birth-weight babies), and as a result, in 1998, the program was expanded to include all Pitney Bowes locations (The Health Project, Inc. 2002).

Areas for Collaboration Between Worksite Health Promotion and Disability Management

¬ Early intervention and provision of wellness programs and fitness resources to promote health

¬ Safety and injury prevention and training for all employees

¬ Job modification to help injured employees return to productive work

¬ Maternity management programs

¬ Enhanced management policies and practices

OCCUPATIONAL HEALTH AND SAFETY

What does occupational health and safety have in common with worksite health promotion? Beyond the compliance and regulatory issues, occupational health and safety managers are concerned with productivity, absenteeism, and workers' compensation costs. Their job is to provide a safe work environment for employees and to keep incidence of injury and lost workdays to a minimum.

In some companies, workers' compensation costs account for approximately 3% of total costs (Barge and Carlson 1993) and injuries account for approximately 15% of unscheduled absences (Goetzel 1998). Therefore, injury prevention, quality medical intervention, and aggressive return-to-work programs become key initiatives in meeting the profitability goals of

the organization. Back injuries, repetitive-strain injuries, and cumulative-trauma injuries represent the most common and most expensive injuries for organizations. These injuries can be minimized or prevented with proper training and education and early intervention. Comprehensive injury prevention and ergonomic programs utilize a cross-functional approach, which includes employee involvement and participation. Components of a good program include training in proper body mechanics, an emphasis on the importance of physical strength and conditioning, sound nutrition, weight management, and smoking cessation. Additionally, researchers have stressed the importance of addressing psychosocial factors, the structure of the work environment, and exposure to hazardous working conditions. Because most occupational health and safety personnel do not have a background in health promotion or fitness and are often more compliance oriented, and because most injuries are a result of human behavior and lifestyle, injury prevention becomes a natural area for collaboration with health promotion professionals.

Champion International Corporation Case Study

At Champion International Corporation, there is a strong belief in and a strategic model for the total health approach in addressing individual needs throughout the continuum of care. Within this model, there is an expectation that the needs of individuals and groups will be met through the partnerships that are developed internally and externally (The Health Project, Inc. 2002). Acting on this expectation, Champion International Corporation initiated an injury prevention and ergonomics program at Nationwide Papers in the early 1990s. They started the process by meeting with the safety teams and general managers to assess the workers' compensation and safety concerns. "We weren't interested in a Band-Aid approach," says Howard Kraft, Manager of Benefits Education and Health Management. Therefore, instead of implementing a traditional classroom-based approach, they took the program to the employees in their offices and in the warehouses. They provided ergonomic assessments and assistance and followed up by educating employees on lifestyle issues, anatomy, physiology, and manual material handling. This innovative program paid off. Champion experienced a 35% decrease in their lost-time accident rate that correlated to savings of $100,000 in workers' compensation costs. "We 'talk the talk and walk the walk'of partnership for all our programs," says Kraft, and "it's paying off."

Mobil Oil Case Study

At Mobil Oil, where there are many small locations with limited staff, such as oil-drilling platforms, the worksite health promotion staff developed simple, easy-to-use programs for supervisors or foremen to implement during their safety meetings. Their programs include a script, video, and handouts. The handouts steer participants to other resources or programs they can access (Cronin 1995).

Union Pacific Railroad Case Study

How do you keep railroad engineers, who are required to work long hours at a control station, from nodding off during their shifts? You let them nap—officially, on company time. At least, this is what Union Pacific Railroad found (Luetzinger, Holland, and Richling 1999). The consequences of drowsiness at work carry huge financial risks for Union Pacific and other transportation companies and can also have significant emergency response implications. It is estimated that fatigue-related expenses can be as much as $2,035 per employee with 35% of these costs attributable to lower performance caused by fatigue. Union Pacific developed a pilot program called SleepWell that was designed to address poor sleep at home and sleepiness at work. The program consisted of a sleep disorders assessment followed by an intervention program called 21 Nights to Better Sleep. In addition to this program, Union Pacific adjusted operational components and work schedules. The estimated cost savings for this group of engineers ranged from $259,000 to $1.25

million. The cost-benefit ratio was calculated to be $3.23:1. Because of these results, Joe Leutzinger, PhD, indicated that "our top management approved the continuation of this program and other fatigue management initiatives."

Areas for Collaboration Between Worksite Health Promotion and Occupational Health and Safety
- Injury prevention
- Ergonomics
- Fatigue management
- Healthy shift work
- Health screenings
- Supervisory training

MEDICAL AND HEALTH SERVICES

Because of the common goals of preventing unnecessary disease and disability and improving quality of life, it is natural for medical and health services and worksite health promotion to integrate their program offerings. Determining what medical conditions to target can be a joint decision based on sharing the results of health risk appraisals or health screenings. Additionally, targeting medical conditions can be further refined by obtaining the results of annual health insurance utilization reviews. With the help of your benefits department and your health insurance provider, you can use aggregate data to determine common lifestyle-related medical conditions that prompt employees to seek out-patient care (e.g., physician or chiropractic office visits) or hospitalization.

In the past, prevention and disease management programs have been focused on prevalent medical conditions such as cardiovascular disease and cancer, but more recently, the scope of medical interventions at the worksite has expanded to include less high-profile but still costly conditions such as osteoporosis, asthma, influenza, and depression. If resources are not available in-house, medical and health services and worksite health promotion can work with the company's health or managed care provider to offer such specialty interventions.

Collaboration between medical and health services and worksite health promotion is often a win-win situation. Referral by the company physician or nurse to the worksite health promotion program can increase the credibility of the health promotion program in the eyes of the employees and reinforce the importance of adopting or maintaining a health-promoting lifestyle. Furthermore, in the case of prevalent occupation-related medical conditions, such as low back injury, medical and health services can team up with occupational health and safety and the worksite health promotion program to provide preinjury screenings, to design exercise programs to prevent and rehabilitate injury, and to offer injury prevention training.

℞ Areas for Collaboration Between Worksite Health Promotion and Medical and Health Services

¬ Influenza vaccination program
¬ Depression management
¬ Diabetes prevention and management
¬ Osteoporosis prevention and management
¬ Asthma management
¬ Self-care (informed health care decision making)
¬ Sponsored mammography campaign

BARRIERS AND CHALLENGES TO INTERNAL ALLIANCES

S Unsettling as it might be to some, out-of-the-box thinking and action can yield remarkable results. Health promotion professionals have a great opportunity to help organizations meet and exceed their business objectives. However, these opportunities do not always seem evident and they sometimes come disguised as threats and problems. The key to successful results stems from an entrepreneurial-type attitude. Operate within a box, and you could be shipped out on the next train. Operate with a solution-oriented approach, and the geese come flocking. Except when they do not. And they do not because of the following reasons:

¬ It is difficult to change the status quo. People, including health promotion professionals, resist change and tend to stick to what they know. Continue to expand your expertise and knowledge into other areas (e.g., strategic planning, disability management, ergonomics, and managed care).

¬ Turf issues are very real, especially when individual job security is threatened. Look for ways to partner with and collaborate with other people and departments. Work to build relationships and develop trust.

¬ There is no shared strategic vision or purpose. This problem may result in miscommunication and lack of follow-through on projects or initiatives. Go back to the drawing board. Agree on goals, objectives, and measurement standards. Define roles and responsibilities. Acquire management approval and involvement.

¬ Integration takes time. Often, health promotion is not on management's radar screen. Don't rush, and begin small. Look for immediate opportunities and build on your successes.

¬ You do not have data or access to the right data sources. This problem results in developing programs and initiatives that may miss the mark completely. Consequently, you do not address the real business needs of the organization. You and your team waste time and resources and decrease your hard-earned credibility.

¬ You operate in numerous locations and report to different decision makers. Having multiple locations and different stakeholders makes for an interesting job. However, your priority is to find out what is bothering them about their employees by utilizing a client-oriented approach. What is the end result? Successful solutions cocreated with your clients.

EXTERNAL ALLIANCES

Over one third of employers outsource some or all of their human resources and benefits programs. This trend continues to climb as large corporations strive to minimize costs and maximize revenues. A survey conducted by the Wellness Program Management Advisor indicated that 93.4% of health promotion professionals use external vendors and consultants for at least a portion of their programs. Furthermore, 73.3% said 1% to 25% of their programs utilize external vendors and consultants, 7% said they use outside vendors and consultants for more than 75% of their program, and 7% said they use outside vendors and consultants for 50% to 75% of their programs (Health Resources Publishing 2002).

Organizations often work closely with vendors to design customized services that will best meet the diverse needs of employees. This approach commonly involves a performance contract that specifies the services to be provided and the costs. Quarterly reviews provide ample opportunity to determine if the services have been provided according to the contract and whether any modifications or adjustments are needed. Examples of common external vendors include

¬ employee assistance programs and work/life consultants;

¬ physicians, hospitals, and managed care organizations;

¬ health promotion product and service vendors;

¬ colleges and universities; and

¬ not-for-profit organizations.

EMPLOYEE ASSISTANCE PROGRAMS AND WORK/LIFE CONSULTANTS

With many health promotion programs now focused on issues that affect not only the health of individuals but also the health of the bottom line, programs that are traditionally offered by employee assistance programs (EAPs) and work/life consultants may now fall under the expanded definition of health promotion. Challenges such as balancing work and family, job insecurity, depression, and substance abuse affect the ability of employees to be fully productive on the job.

Employee problems and concerns are most commonly a result of several issues, and the solution can cross several functional boundaries. For instance, an employee who is going through a divorce may not be the ideal candidate to begin an exercise program. Likewise, an individual who is experiencing depression because he or she has diabetes may need health counseling in conjunction with EAP counseling.

Depression Case Study

A multinational financial institution started a depression awareness and education program after benefit claims from pharmacies uncovered the disturbing fact that antidepressants were the number one medication prescribed to their employees. EAP utilization had also increased. This effort has resulted in a successful collaboration involving worksite health promotion staff, EAP providers, work/life consultants, benefits administrators, and physicians. In the last quarter of 1998, the company offered a voluntary, confidential depression-screening program called ETAP (Employee Telephone Access Program) developed by the National Depression Screening Project, in which all calls were anonymous. In addition, EAP providers were brought on site to provide depression awareness programs as well. The services were promoted through the use of posters, brochures, newsletter articles, payroll stuffers, and displays at the various locations and by worksite health promotion staff. The next phase of the depression awareness program involved aggressive outreach to physicians (who are prescribing antidepressants to employees) to educate them on treatment guidelines. In addition, the company provided outreach to employees who had mental health claims or existing diseases where depression is a common issue (The Health Project, Inc. 2002).

PHYSICIANS, HOSPITALS, AND MANAGED CARE ORGANIZATIONS

The integration of worksite health promotion and community-based medical services depends on the development of partnerships among physicians, hospitals, managed care organizations, and insurance carriers. Through such partnerships, primary (prevention of onset of disease), secondary (early detection of disease), and tertiary (management of advanced disease to prevent disability) care can be linked. Through such partnerships, a worksite health promotion program can identify what health care services are available so as not to duplicate programs and cost. Additionally, interfacing the worksite program with medical providers in community-based or managed care–based settings can be an important means of increasing employee participation in worksite health promotion programs and referrals of high-risk employees from physicians to worksite programs.

Coronary Bypass Surgery
Case Study

Physicians with patients returning to work after coronary bypass surgery collaborated with health promotion professionals in the Stanford University worksite wellness program to coordinate the aftercare of their patients. In particular, in conjunction with the physicians, the worksite health promotion program developed a plan for monitoring the employees' physiological status at work, facilitating their compliance with health behavior–related therapeutic regimens, and encouraging them to develop and maintain health-promoting behaviors. Reciprocally, the worksite health promotion program identified high-risk employees through implementation of routine health risk appraisals and screenings and referred them to community-based or health plan–affiliated physicians (Stokols, Pelletier, and Fielding 1995).

Duke University Case Study

Duke University has also instituted linkages between physicians and the University's Live for Life worksite health promotion program. The Live for Life program encourages physicians to refer high-risk patients to the worksite health promotion program. High-risk employees are identified by occupational health physicians overseeing job-related-injury recovery programs and preplacement physical examinations and by primary care physicians in the course of delivering routine medical care. In addition, the Live for Life program also encourages physicians to include health promotion services in their summary reports, recommendations, and health prescriptions (Kenny and Jackson 1998).

HealthPartners Case Study

Linkage between medical care providers and worksite health promotion programs can also be initiated by health care organizations. In 1995, HealthPartners, a non-profit, consumer-governed group of health care organizations, originated the Partners of Better Health Employer Initiative. The purpose of the initiative is to improve organizational and employee health in Minnesota by reducing the total burden and total cost of illness. Because the group recognized that such health-related goals are difficult to attain by any one entity, four key stakeholder entities work collaboratively: HealthPartner organizations, clinical providers, employers, and employees who are members of a HealthPartner organization (Pronk and Entzion 1998).

HEALTH PROMOTION SPECIALTY PRODUCT AND SERVICE VENDORS

A common model in organizations that provide health promotion services is to maintain a core group of health promotion staff that plans and implements the program, while purchasing various products and services from other companies. For instance, in-house staff may run the corporate fitness center, yet purchase health-risk appraisal (also called health-risk assessment or HRA) services and educational resources from an outside vendor. Larger organizations may outsource several functions, including HRA services, medical self-care programs, a prenatal program, and nurse triage services. Still other companies have chosen to outsource the entire corporate health promotion program. These organizations have made the determination that they obtain a better program at a lower cost, thereby gaining a better value. In the long run, to outsource this human resource function not only reduces the organizations' head counts but also allows them to focus on their core business competencies.

Types of Health Promotion Specialty Product and Service Vendors

¬ Facility design and management services

¬ Health-risk appraisal administration and analysis services

¬ Disease management services

¬ Nurse advice and triage services

¬ Prenatal products and services

¬ Medical self-care products and services

¬ Educational products and services

Texas Instruments Case Study

Whether an organization outsources part or all of its health promotion functions, the programs must be tied to the organization's business needs and objectives. One organization that outsourced several key health promotion services but maintained a core health promotion staff was Texas Instruments (TI). Marsha McCabe, former health promotion manager at TI, shared the process that TI utilized to choose and manage vendors who provided health care services to TI's then more than 43,000 employees. TI initially developed a philosophical framework for the kinds of vendors they would consider. For instance, TI insisted that selected vendors utilize the stage of readiness model and provide a high degree of customer service. As services from a vendor were needed, TI would disseminate a request for proposal (RFP). The RFP would provide vendors with clear guidelines and criteria that outlined the critical success factors by which they would be judged. On completion of the RFP process and selection of a vendor, TI drew up a performance contract that would delineate the agreed-upon program outcomes that the vendor would be held accountable for.

Many vendors provide a comprehensive menu of services to clients, including fitness center management, screening and assessment, injury prevention, health education programs, and disease management. Other vendors have developed niche products and specialize in a certain area or product. For instance, 10 years ago, there were only a handful of companies providing health risk appraisal services. Today, there is a myriad of vendors listed in the Society for Prospective Medicine's guidebook, demonstrating the growth in the market. Likewise, in the demand management as well as in the disease management areas, there are a variety of programs and strategies developed to help organizations manage the health and health care costs of their population.

FACILITY DESIGN AND MANAGEMENT SERVICES

Nowadays, an organization can contract from several companies that have in-depth experi-

ence and expertise in planning and running corporate fitness centers. Fitness center vendors may provide the following services:

¬ Feasibility studies
¬ Facility design and development
¬ Equipment selection
¬ Staff hiring and training
¬ Development and implementation of operating systems (e.g., participation tracking, financial planning and budgeting, marketing and promotion, and behavior change strategies)
¬ Day-to-day program administration

HEALTH-RISK APPRAISAL ADMINISTRATION AND ANALYSIS SERVICES

HRAs can be a valuable resource for health promotion professionals in designing, implementing, and evaluating their programs. There are a number of assessment tools available with various features and optional components. The primary objectives of an HRA are to

¬ identify the overall health status and health risks of the population;
¬ identify at-risk individuals or those with chronic conditions; and
¬ measure change in outcomes over time.

In addition to meeting these primary objectives, many HRA programs provide an intervention component that may include personalized health reports for participants that identify specific action items to reduce risk, health education materials, and telephonic outreach to at-risk individuals. These interventions serve to reinforce behavior change over time.

A more recent development in HRA programs is an emphasis on individuals with chronic conditions or who are at risk for becoming high medical care utilizers. For many health promotion professionals beginning to address this issue, an HRA that identifies and provides interventions for at-risk populations is a valuable resource. One size does not fit all in the HRA industry. Many professionals want a tool they can use in-house as is, but others want full customization options. Some want to add other data sources such as participation or fitness center utilization, whereas others are looking for a tool that can demonstrate a return on investment. It is the responsibility of the health promotion professional to shop around and find a tool or to modify a tool already on the market to meet his or her specific needs.

DISEASE MANAGEMENT SERVICES

Many health promotion professionals are beginning to expand their reach to individuals with or at risk for chronic disease. This relatively new and evolving field provides a significant potential for worksite health promotion programs to address the needs of individuals throughout the entire health care continuum—from a state of positive health to chronic disease. Some health promotion programs are utilizing HRA and telephonic services to serve this population. Some of the services these external vendors provide include the following:

¬ Identification of at-risk individuals. Some vendors utilize an assessment (e.g., HRA), whereas others identify high-risk individuals using health insurance utilization data.

¬ Interventions. This component may include successive assessments with follow-up health reports and health education materials, outbound calls made by registered nurses or health educators, and self-directed materials.

¬ Evaluation. This component generally includes self-reported health risk, behavior change, or health insurance utilization data.

Chevron Case Study

D'Ann Whitehead, Preventive Health Services Manager at Chevron, indicated that the company's expectation at each location is to utilize existing health care resources. A health promotion staff person is responsible for coordinating the services offered by the local health plans and pharmaceutical firms. Chevron's strategy is to target programs by analyzing health risk, behavior change, and health insurance utilization data and look for matches. The next step is to find out what programs are in place and then, in collaboration with the health care companies, target one or two areas. "Focus on only one or two areas. Otherwise the [health plans] won't deliver."

NURSE ADVICE AND TRIAGE SERVICES

Nurse advice and triage services is a round-the-clock service that typically provides a wealth of computerized health care information and telephone lines to registered nurses or other trained medical personnel. Their job is to help individuals determine their condition, its seriousness, the appropriate self-care and treatment options, and how soon treatment should be sought. Although a trained nurse can offer comfort and advice to an anxious parent whose child has a high fever or direct a caller with chest pain to the emergency room, they specifically do not diagnose. Rather, they use medically designed, detailed, peer-reviewed triage protocols gleaned from medical literature to assess symptoms, determine the seriousness, give advice, and support the callers in making their own decisions about their medical care.

Nurse advice and triage services is rapidly expanding because so much medical utilization is considered unnecessary. For example, it has been reported that as much as 60% of all primary care visits are unnecessary and 50% of all emergency room visits do not involve urgent care (McCarthy 1997). Obviously, therein lies an enormous opportunity to save a significant amount of health care dollars and at the same time help individuals become better medical-care consumers.

A significant number of self-insured and managed care companies now offer nurse advice and triage services to its employees or members. It is usually free to members and is available 24 hours a day, 7 days a week, 365 days a year. Many worksite health promotion program managers may be involved in developing the performance contract and may be involved in ongoing management activities with the vendor. Usually companies that provide this service are eager to work with health promotion program staff to design promotional packages and conduct ongoing marketing activities to increase utilization.

PRENATAL PRODUCTS AND SERVICES

Maternal and infant health is an area that demands attention from corporate executives and the worksite health program staff alike. Women are entering the workforce in tremendous numbers; thus, there is great need to develop corporate-sponsored maternity and family-care programs. Additionally, childbirth-related costs may represent the largest health care expenditure for organizations. From 10% to 49% of annual health care costs are attributable to maternity cases, according to the Bureau of National Affairs. A single birth can cost anywhere from $20,000 to $250,000 (Jacobson, Kolarek, and Newton 1996). The opportunity for employers is tremendous. Much of the cost is related to lifestyle factors under the control of the parents and is, therefore, preventable. For instance, the New York Lung Association estimates that 22% of low-birth-weight babies are attributable to smoking.

The results of worksite prenatal health education programs are overwhelmingly positive, demonstrating reduced numbers of low-birth-weight babies and unnecessary cesarean sections, shorter hospital stays, fewer days in intensive care, and less absenteeism. The added benefit is that the organization creates a nurturing partnership with their employees who are starting families. Many worksite programs turn to external vendors to provide a prenatal health education program for their population. Generally, the program provides successive risk assessments with outreach for women identified as being at risk. These assessments may be tied to each trimester and may be delivered through the mail, electronically, or over the telephone.

> The challenge for health promotion professionals is promoting the services to their populations. Announcements and testimonials in newsletters, posters, and brochures serve to remind eligible women about the service. Another challenge is integrating the program with the woman's medical service. Educating the physician population may be a challenge but will be well worth the effort.

Personalized letters and educational booklets that provide support and health education information are typically used. A book such as *What to Expect When You're Expecting* may be included as well. Some programs offer a 24-hour information line and prerecorded health information messages.

Evaluation of the program is usually derived from a postpartum questionnaire that asks for information about the woman's birth outcomes. For instance, did the woman have a cesarean section or did she deliver vaginally? How much did the baby weigh? Were there any medical problems? Because health claims data are frequently difficult to obtain, these outcome measures provide valuable information in determining the success of the program.

MEDICAL SELF-CARE PRODUCTS AND SERVICES

Medical self-care (MSC) is rapidly becoming the cornerstone of every health promotion program that is interested in reducing health care costs. Multiple research studies have demonstrated the effectiveness of MSC programs. On average, 17% of outpatient visits are avoided after the implementation of an effective MSC program. Furthermore, individuals report having more confidence about knowing how to treat minor medical problems as a result of an MSC program (Vickery et al. 1983). MSC programs educate individuals on how to manage their medical symptoms in the most effective way and how to use the medical-care system more appropriately. MSC programs typically include an MSC book paired with an initial training program that gives participants experience in using the book. The MSC book guides the individual with minor symptoms to home treatment and self-care and guides those with more significant problems to further assessment and treatment. MSC serves as an effective first step in changing behaviors. Furthermore, it provides an immediate (first-year) return on investment with its well-rounded approach to total wellness.

EDUCATIONAL PRODUCTS AND SERVICES

Years ago, health promotion professionals needed to be savvy program developers and to possess a creative spirit to design promotional pieces (e.g., newsletters) for high impact. Nowadays, health promotion programs can choose from the myriad of educational resources available that can meet their budget and program development needs such as newsletters, self-directed behavior change programs, educational brochures, software, incentive programs, brown bag seminars, external vendors, and consultants. The most prevalent use of external educational resources, as cited in a 1998 study conducted by Wellness Program Advisor, is the purchase of "wellness kits." External vendors were used for this purpose by 71% of survey respondents. An additional 29% used external vendors for staffing, class instruction, and brown bag seminars. Other respondents indicated they looked to organizations such as Wellness Councils of America (WELCOA), a national nonprofit organization dedicated to promotion of healthy workplaces, to just "get ideas" (Health Resources Publishing 2002). Clearly, health promotion programs can tap into the growing market of health care information sources to provide some or a majority of their health care educational needs.

UNIVERSITIES AND COLLEGES

Institutions of higher education can augment worksite health promotion programs by providing free or low-cost consulting, manpower resources, employee training, and facilities. Faculty affiliated with local universities or colleges frequently provide consultation services for worksite health promotion program design and evaluation. Additionally, as part of their research, they sometimes plan, implement, and evaluate custom-made comprehensive health promotion programs. Computer information systems faculty develop and test database management systems. If faculty do not deliver services directly, their students often do so as part of a course requirement (internship, practicum, or field experience class) or on a volunteer basis. Such services can include health screening assessment, fitness assessment and exercise program development, behavior change incentive programs, health promotion educational sessions, and health promotion displays.

Furthermore, university faculty and students sometimes provide on-site health promotion seminar series or workshops. Sometimes, the university will partner with local health care providers such as public health departments and managed care organizations to provide paraprofessional training to companies interested in starting a worksite health promotion program (Golaszewski, Barr, and Cochran 1998).

Finally, institutions of higher education sometimes provide tuition and fee discounts to employees of companies that utilize the uni-

versity or college as an outsource provider for their worksite health promotion program. Such an arrangement can be a win-win situation for both the institution of higher education and the company. The revenue generated from facility membership fees, program participation fees, or tuition allows universities and colleges to upgrade facilities and hire staff that in turn can offer state-of-the-art programs to company employees at a discounted cost (King 1997).

PHILANTHROPIC ORGANIZATIONS

Budgets are tight, resources are limited, yet worksite health promotion managers are expected to meet the diverse health needs of their employees. Fortunately, there is a wealth of information and resources available for those who proactively search. Philanthropic organizations, the programs they offer, and their Web site addresses are listed in the sidebar.

Programs Offered by Philanthropic Organizations

Heart at Work Program
American Heart Association
www.americanheart.org

American Lung Association
www.lungusa.org

March of Dimes Foundation
www.modimes.org

National Institute on Alcohol Abuse and Alcoholism Publications/Databases
www.niaaa.nih.gov

National Mental Health Association
www.nmha.org

American Dietetic Association
www.eatright.org

Heart at Work Program

Often, health promotion professionals look for "wellness kits" to supplement their program offerings. The Heart at Work Program, offered by the American Heart Association, is an excellent tool for staff with limited budgets and time commitments. Heart disease claims more 550,000 lives annually and is the leading cause of death in the United States and other developed countries. Much of this disease is preventable through proper attention to risk factors such as elevated blood lipids, hypertension, cigarette smoking, physical inactivity, obesity, diabetes mellitus, diet, and tension and stress. The Heart at Work Program focuses on the personal health practices that are vital and paramount to decreasing the risk of heart disease (Chambers 1995). The program includes

¬ a Program Coordinator's Guide, which is a comprehensive resource for planning and implementing the activity modules provided;

¬ periodically enhanced and updated modules that cover a variety of heart-healthy topics such as heart attack assessments, blood pressure, cholesterol, physical activity, and cessation of tobacco use; and

¬ optional on-site training and videos that provide comprehensive assistance.

BARRIERS AND CHALLENGES TO EXTERNAL ALLIANCES

Howard Kraft at Champion International indicated that the biggest challenge they face with their outside providers is keeping everyone focused on the common interests of all parties, which is to enhance the health and well-being of employees and their dependents. Providers may be competing for business elsewhere and may therefore be reluctant to work together. However, when the expectation of cooperation is clearly communicated and stipulated in the performance contracts, there is an incentive for partnering and collaboration.

At Texas Instruments (TI), they utilized a number of vendors to provide important services to employees and their dependents to enhance health and well-being. Marsha McCabe at TI provided the following list of challenges they faced while dealing with vendors who provided services for 43,000 employees and their dependents.

¬ Communication with the end-user (employees and dependents) and with vendors. The programs and services are only effective if individuals utilize the service, so the focus is always on increasing visibility and utilization. After the initial launch period, worksite health promotion staff may not have the opportunity to continually promote the program. Therefore, the staff needs to rely on the internal cross-referrals from the vendors and the communications infrastructure

developed at the company. In the past, the TI staff met once a year with all providers to share information and build rapport. This procedure proved to be difficult because there was constant turnover with providers that required a re-education process. Now TI electronically updates its vendors on a regular basis. For instance, when they added a new feature (e.g., depression screening), it was critical for all the vendors to know about the new service and when and how to refer individuals to it.

¬ Seamless integration of services. TI faced this challenge by providing multiple delivery channels (e.g., on-site, printed materials, intranet and e-mail, and telephone) for easy access. They also made their providers accountable for providing cross-referrals. It was stipulated in the performance contract that, in addition to providing outcome statistics on the service (e.g., how many emergency room visits were avoided), vendors had to indicate how many referrals were made to the other providers. Obviously, this information needed to be constantly updated. Their nurse line service had a brief description of all the related health vendors, including the key contacts and hours of operation. Another example of TI's effort to make the operation seamless among vendors involved their smoking cessation initiative. Participants who wanted to receive a nicotine patch were required to be enrolled in a smoking cessation program. The smoking cessation vendor was required to notify the pharmacy of who was enrolled.

¬ Technology and information. The first challenge is to collect the data and then turn them into information. After that, the challenge is to turn the information into knowledge. "This is where technology will change the landscape in the future," says Marsha. There is a constant challenge to educate and inform managers and key decision makers in a compelling way about the value of the programs. Integration of data will be critical to meeting this challenge. Even at TI, where technology is robust, the services and statistics are not integrated into a total package. Therefore, it is difficult to understand the total benefit delivered by each service.

SUMMARY

As models and theories are strongly related, examination and comprehension of one or all of the models and theories described here provide a strong foundation for the planning process that is followed. A planning process that has its roots in accepted theory provides the underpinnings for a successful program that achieves the outcomes desired by all the parties involved. In addition, effective planning involves both in-house and out-of-house partners whose expertise is complementary in nature to allow for division of labor. Some possible partners include employees, work teams, the organization with its customers, vendors, shareholders, the community, and government entities.

REFERENCES

Barge, B., and J. Carlson. 1993. *Controlling health care and disability costs*. New York: Wiley.

Cash, G. 1997. Financial wellness: Your next health promotion program. *Worksite Health* 4:20-22.

Cavanaugh, K., and M. Yarborough. 1996. Vanderbilt integrates health promotion and human resources. *Worksite Health* 3:14-21.

Chambers, C. 1995. New Heart at Work Program offers something for everyone. *Worksite Health* 2:30-31.

Cronin, C. 1995. Partner with occupational health and safety to extend your reach. *Worksite Health* 2:29-30.

Goetzel, R. 1998. Proceedings of AWHP 1998 International Conference: Productivity and health management: Benchmarking of an emerging paradigm in worksite health management.

Golaszewski, T., D. Barr, and S. Cochran. 1998. Teaming up with academia: The vendors' fair revisited. *Worksite Health* 5:15-17.

Health Resources Publishing. (2002). *Wellness Junction*. Available: www.wellnessjunction.com.

Jacoboon, M., M. Kolarek, and B. Newton, 1996. *Business, babies and the bottom line: Corporate innovations and best practices in maternal and child health*. Washington, DC: Washington Business Group on Health.

Kenny, G.M., and G.W. Jackson. 1998. Duke's Wellness Program successfully partners with physicians. *Worksite Health* 5:13-15.

King, L. 1997. Community memberships support university-based program. *Worksite Health* 4:36-39.

Leutzinger, J.A., D.W. Holland, and D.E. Richling. 1999. Good moon rising: Union Pacific Railroad's Alertness-Management Program. *Worksite Health* 6:16-20.

McCarthy, R. 1997. It takes more than a phone to manage demand. *Business and Health* 15:36-41.

Pronk, N.D., and K. Entzion. 1998. Worksite health promotion and managed care: Creating partnerships for population health improvement. *Worksite Health* 5:10-17.

Stokols, D., Pelletier, K.R., and J.E. Fielding. 1995. Integration of medical care and worksite health promotion. *Journal of the American Medical Association* 273:1136-1142.

The Health Project, Inc. 2002. Employer health register. www.healthproject.stanford.edu.

Vickery, D.M., H. Kalmer, D. Lowry, M. Constantine, E. Wright, and W. Loren. 1983. Effect of a self-care education program on medical visits. *Journal of the American Medical Association* 250:2952-2956.

Part I Summary

From the CEO's perspective, reaching into the true potential of people within organizations may only be facilitated in an environment that is freely willing to incorporate healthy behaviors, beliefs, attitudes, and values into its daily operations.

A cycle of planning, implementation, and evaluation results in a highly integrated program that brings about specific health behavior changes that ultimately lead to the outcomes desired by an organization. Frequently, however, these worksite health promotion programs are designed and implemented in isolation from other departments within a company.

Integration of both internal and external resources, coupled with out-of-the-box thinking and action, spurs remarkable results. Now and in the future, properly trained and qualified health promotion professionals have an impressive opportunity to help organizations meet and exceed their business objectives.

Part II

Operation Processes That Work

Part Objectives

Purpose

- ¬ To provide readers with the information required to establish and administer a health promotion initiative that meets the needs and goals of the organization being served
- ¬ To provide readers with a written resource tool useful in the development and operation of a best-practice health promotion program
- ¬ To assist readers in developing health promotion programs that achieve measurable outcomes

Application

- ¬ An understanding of the customer's "customer" leads to the development and ongoing operation of health promotion programs that meet the needs and goals of the organization being served.
- ¬ Suggestions for identifying and utilizing the most appropriate and advantageous resources are provided, maximizing the potential for program efficiency and cost benefit.
- ¬ A planning and implementation process is recommended so that program development and operations can occur in a productive manner.
- ¬ Appropriate interventions are recommended, and how they may be integrated with other elements of the health promotion program and other health-related services within the organization is discussed. Best-practice examples are also provided.
- ¬ Operating pitfalls to avoid such as liability, legal concerns, and staff turnover are discussed.

Vision

- ¬ The four cornerstones to an effective health promotion program are needs assessment and evaluation, healthy culture development, effective interventions, and relapse prevention. Each cornerstone has a unique relationship to the other three, and all four must be developed effectively for the health promotion program to be maximally successful.

Chapter 4

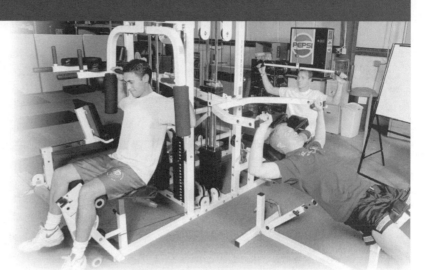

Establishing the Operating Plan and Resources

The operating plan may be the most important element of a successful health promotion program. Once the benefits of health promotion at the worksite, in the community, and in our personal lives is understood, the question is not whether to provide a health promotion program but how we do it. In this section we will provide the "how-to" steps to success by addressing management practices and operational processes professionals need when developing and building successful health promotion programs.

There is no single formula for operating successful health promotion programs. Presented throughout this manual are models and processes that are working within various settings. Although a program for a Fortune 500 company with multiple locations worldwide may look very different from the program at a company with fewer than 50 employees at a single location, the overall components for success are similar. These components include four cornerstones: (1) needs assessment and evaluation, (2) healthy culture development, (3) effective interventions, and (4) relapse prevention.

While the focus of this book is on worksite health promotion, it is impossible to exclude other settings and environments when addressing overall health promotion. The reality is that a small corporation with fewer than 50 employees may rely on the YMCA, a commercial health club, or the hospital down the street to provide cost-effective, relatively convenient and beneficial health promotion services for its employees. These organizations may also provide valuable opportunities for family members and retirees who otherwise might be excluded from an on-site corporate program.

> What is different in each setting are the delivery methods and systems and, of course, the resources available. The key is to evaluate and coordinate the available resources and to apply those resources to an agreed-upon mission and goals.

One of the challenges in part II is to include both facility-based and non–facility-based programs in the overview of operations. It is impossible to exclude facility-based programs if we are to recognize and highlight the importance of physical activity in our definition of health promotion. A fitness or wellness center that includes exercise equipment often provides the platform for program delivery even though such equipment is not a necessity or even affordable for many organizations. A physical fitness facility can be a key avenue for supporting health enhancement, disease management, disability management, and incentive programs, but these programs can also be supported in the absence of a physical facility. Thus, an attempt has been made to show how program development and operation should occur, both when physical facilities are available and when they are not.

UNDERSTANDING THE CUSTOMER

When implementing a worksite health promotion operation, understanding the customer is essential. The following is a process that can serve as a guide for understanding the needs of the customer.

ORGANIZATIONAL GOALS AND OBJECTIVES

To receive and maintain support, health promotion initiatives must be consistent with and support the goals and objectives of the organization being served. Often, the general focus of the corporate customer is described in the company's mission statement. The business and strategic plans provide a more detailed description of the direction of the organization. Finally, the specific goals and objectives of the organization and each department provide the most definitive description of what the organization is attempting to accomplish, especially in the immediate future. The health promotion professional must be thoroughly familiar with this information and design programs that will contribute to the overall business success of the customer.

ORGANIZATIONAL DEMOGRAPHICS AND CULTURE

For health promotion initiatives to be successful, they must be appropriate for the demographics and culture of the organization. Demographics such as average age of the population, age stratification, gender mix, ethnic mix, and employee type (i.e., active versus retiree or salaried versus hourly) are all factors that help determine what types of programs are most appropriate for the population.

Cultural factors such as the psychographic composition and the geographic composition of the organization are also important in implementing the most efficacious program. Psychographic components include factors such as the prevailing attitudes, level of organizational support, current morale, and trust within the organization. Tools are available to audit the culture and even determine if support exists for health promotion activities. Geographic factors include the geographical dispersion of the persons to be served and the transience of this population.

An important cultural factor to consider is whether the organization is unionized. If it is unionized, meeting the mission and needs of the union and the company, without negatively affecting one or the other, is an additional challenge that must be met.

By implementing health promotion programs that meet both the demographic and cultural needs, the potential for success is maximized.

ORGANIZATIONAL STRUCTURE AND PATTERNS

Knowing the customer and providing the most applicable health promotion services requires a thorough understanding of the organizational structure and change patterns. The work environment (i.e., manufacturing site, headquarters operation, sales force, or mixed-use environment) to some extent drives the organizational structure, but sweeping changes are occurring in organizational development. After more than 50 years of the functional hierarchy or pyramidal organization, most companies are moving to a more flat or horizontal organization. Such a structure involves integrated work teams, participative management, cross-trained employees, and a focus on having persons performing related tasks working together.

The operating structure of the organization is a significant factor in the delivery of health promotion at the worksite. The planning and delivery of health promotion programs must be consistent with the organizational structure and thus include the correct level of employee involvement. Additionally, support must be received from a series of smaller units, with greater interpersonal support, motivation, and empowerment to act. In knowing the customer, health promotion professionals must learn the nuances of the structure and endeavor to work within it effectively.

ORGANIZATIONAL INTEGRATION

To understand your customer, you must be informed about how the organization is integrated and how the health promotion program fits into the existing structure. Often, the health promotion staff reports to the human resources department, benefits office, medical services, corporate services, or occupational health. Regardless of where health promotion staff report, integration with other departments is essential. Any of the departments listed previously can support the health promotion mission. In addition, departments such as organizational development, corporate planning, finance, and marketing and communications can be important allies. These groups can lend expertise to the health promotion effort, and the health promotion effort can in turn significantly influence their missions, business plans, goals, and objectives.

⌐P̶ *Customer Service Checklist*

¬ Assess the corporate, division, and department mission statements.

¬ Assess the corporate, division, and department business plans.

¬ Assess the corporate, division, and department goals and objectives.

¬ Assess the corporate, division, and department strategic plan.

¬ Assess the culture, demographics, psychographics, and geographics of the organization and its divisions and departments.

¬ Learn the organizational structure and how to work within it.

¬ Integrate with other areas in the organization, both to receive additional expertise and to have them embrace and support the health promotion initiative as part of their business solutions.

¬ Understand the "buying motives" of both decision makers and decision influencers.

RESOURCE AND ALLIANCE UTILIZATION

R̶ (I) Once the customer is understood, the potential resources available for the development and delivery of the health promotion program must be determined. The amount of resources available will influence the eventual operating plan. Health promotion departments are usually small and often have limited budgets. Additionally, their mission is often to create a return on investment. As a result, it is essential that health promotion professionals seek opportunities to deliver high-quality, efficacious, cost-effective programs. Often this effort will involve collaboration with a combination of free and at-cost services. When the business

plan is developed for the health promotion program, and once the plan is reconciled against the budget, the resources and alliances that will be utilized to carry out the plan can be identified.

Resources include people, products, and services that can be utilized in the health promotion initiative. They may be free or available at a cost. Alliances may be established with organizations that share a common interest in the health promotion mission, can derive benefit from it, and can contribute to its accomplishment. In an alliance, the health promotion department and its partner work closely together to achieve mutually beneficial results.

In seeking the resources necessary to carry out the health promotion initiative and in identifying any appropriate alliance partners, the health promotion professional should look within the organization being served, to its health plans, to the community, and to external vendors.

R̶ *Consider the following when seeking internal resources or alliances:*

¬ The corporate communications office can often provide avenues for "advertising" health promotion programs and events. Possibilities include existing newsletters, bulletin boards, corporate e-mail, or voice mail.

¬ The finance department can often provide recommendations for evaluating the cost-benefit ratio or cost-effectiveness.

¬ The corporate planning or organizational development department can assist with long-range planning.

¬ The benefits department may be able to provide funding or resources for communications on health-related issues.

¬ The medical department can sometimes provide facilities, materials, or effective advertising.

¬ Senior management or union leadership can provide a company-wide message supporting the program or a specific event.

¬ *Internal alliances:* The benefits department is often an appropriate group with which to affiliate. This department has a vested interest in controlling health care costs and improving the overall well-being of employees, retirees, and dependents. The benefits department also has the ability to effectively communicate to all of these constituencies.

¬ The medical department often has a mission akin to health promotion. The health promotion staff can assist persons with specific behavioral needs who are referred by the medical staff. Likewise, persons identified through the health promotion program as having specific medical needs can be referred to the medical department. The medical department is also a good venue for distribution of various types of health promotion information. Both parties can work together to affect the well-being of employees.

¬ Labor unions can be excellent alliance partners for delivering health promotion initiatives. Unions are concerned with the health of their members and often negotiate with employers for better health programs. They have credibility among their members and a major voice in how the overall company operates. Union leaders are elected and, like most politicians, want their membership to be aware of the programs they have helped implement. However, as a cautionary note, health promotion professionals must not become too closely aligned with either union or management so as not to alienate one party or the other.

¬ The human resources department in general and, often more specifically, the organizational development staff is charged with creating an environment in which workers function productively with commitment and a sense of well-being. The health promotion department can help them accomplish this task. An alliance with the human resources department or the organizational development staff can be valuable for all parties, and sometimes the health promotion department can draw from the larger budgets possessed by these more mainstream departments.

¬ Most companies have a department such as employee services, which manages health club and other recreational activities. The health promotion department can work in alliance with the employee services department to support health-oriented activities (i.e., walking, running, or cooking). In turn, the employee services department supports health promotion by funding club and other health-oriented events.

HEALTH PLANS

[R] [I] Employers have four choices when considering using their health care plans to deliver some (or all) of their health promotion program. (1) They can do nothing and hope that health care costs do not increase and

that the health of their employees stays stable. (2) They can operate their own health promotion programs, thus fully controlling their own destiny. (3) They can transfer their responsibility for preventing disease to their health plans and hope the providers do a good job. (4) They can share the responsibility with their health plans. This fourth option is often a strategy that is efficacious and cost-efficient for both parties.

Health plans have a health promotion dilemma. On one hand, as employers agree to more managed care capitated arrangements (thus assuming more financial risk), there is an incentive to prevent disease through health promotion. On the other hand, as costs become more tightly controlled, it is difficult for them to spare the resources necessary to provide effective health promotion services, especially given that the return on investment is often several years away. Therefore, if health plans are to be used as a resource in the delivery of worksite health promotion programs, their services must be chosen carefully with attention to quality assurance. The health promotion professional must also recognize that these services may not be delivered cost free.

Services that health plans can sometimes provide include the following:

¬ Health-risk assessments

¬ Targeted health interventions such as disease management, high-risk interventions, case management, or staged mailings

¬ Consumerism assistance such as nurse lines, medical self-care, and audio health libraries

¬ Health promotion classes or seminars

COMMUNITY

[R] [I] Community services can be of value when delivering worksite health promotion programs. Not-for-profit agencies such as the American Red Cross, the American Heart Association, and the American Diabetes Association can provide valuable services, including both professional expertise and appropriate materials and support products.

Local hospitals also can be of service. Often hospitals can be a cost-efficient source of health screenings, seminars, and other general health promotion services. Finally, local professionals such as doctors, nurses, and dieticians will sometimes provide their expertise on request. The use of community resources and alliances in the delivery of worksite health promotion programs is a viable means of receiving valuable expertise and assistance, often at a reasonable cost.

VENDORS

R I Over the past 15 years, there has been an evolution from most employee-based health promotion programs being delivered by in-house staff to a considerable number of programs now being provided by outside vendors. While outside vendors may not know the environment of the worksite as well as on-site staff, it is their responsibility to learn about and assimilate into the culture. Some advantages of using health promotion vendors are as follows:

¬ They bring a global knowledge, having worked with a variety of entities and cultures.

¬ The vendor's sole focus is the delivery of health promotion. Often persons delivering health promotion in-house also have other job assignments.

¬ They often have sophisticated tools and programs, given that they can spread the cost across many clients.

¬ Vendors may have better reach to a company's geographically dispersed workforce.

¬ Often vendors are less expensive than the cost of in-house professionals and easier to eliminate if necessary.

An important task in utilizing vendors as resources or alliances is choosing those with the capabilities required to perform the work and who can consistently deliver high-quality services that result in the appropriate outcomes. See appendix 1 for a guide for selecting vendors (Harris, McKenzie, and Zuti 2002).

SELECTING THE PRIMARY PROGRAM MANAGEMENT APPROACH

R I Rarely are worksite health promotion programs provided solely by in-house professionals or solely by external resources. Instead, programs are usually delivered by a combination of internal and external resources. Programs range from being primarily delivered by in-house staff to being primarily delivered by external providers. Health promotion programs can be successful regardless of where they fall on this continuum, but when planning the program a decision must be made as to how the program will be operated. Often, this decision will be based on what you are trying to achieve, the management approach preferable in the corporate culture, and the resources available.

If employees within the organization are the primary providers of health promotion services, they must meet the specific needs of their "internal" customers. While employees inside the organization often have a first-hand understanding of organizational needs, they must continually be concerned about maintaining a global perspective and staying abreast of new developments within the field.

If services are being provided by entities external to the organization, the professionals involved will have less firsthand knowledge of the customer's needs and thus must gather more information. While this requirement may be an initial handicap, external organizations can bring a global perspective and a number of unique programs and resources.

When developing the operating plan, the management approach to be utilized should be carefully determined and should remain open to flexibility as the program evolves with time. Following are different management approaches that could be chosen.

INTEGRATED MANAGEMENT APPROACH

R I The best approach for many organizations may be a delivery model that involves some services being provided by in-house personnel; some services contracted to third-party vendors; and some services requiring specialized facilities, equipment, and personnel provided off-site by outside organizations such as local hospitals, commercial fitness and health clubs, community resources, and health plan providers.

41

Many best-practice organizations, those "best-in-class" with documented successful programs, are taking the more integrated and strategic approach to managing health promotion programs. This team management approach uses a broad range of resources including internal staff, outside vendors, and health care professionals.

In 1997, the American Productivity and Quality Centers Institute and the MEDSTAT Group, a consulting firm based in Ann Arbor, Michigan, completed a study examining best practices in health and productivity management. Using an interdisciplinary team approach and effective use of internal and external resources were both sited as strategies used by best-practice organizations (Elliott 1998).

In-House Programs

Many organizations choose to develop and operate their health promotion programs using primarily internal resources. There are some excellent in-house programs operating today and, in fact, some organizations see in-house programs as the preferable method of delivery.

When the health promotion staff are full-time employees, they often have a larger stake in the overall success of the program. These employees are recognized as colleagues within the workplace and often have better access to internal resources such as occupational health and safety, maintenance, security, human resources, and other corporate departments. These relationships can foster a more integrated cross-functional approach to service delivery.

Staff salaries are typically higher for in-house health promotion professionals. A 1997 study (Association for Worksite Health Promotion 1997) compared a cross section of the salaries paid to professionals within the health promotion, wellness, and fitness industry. The survey looked at two basic position categories: project management and prescriptive exercise and health promotion. Positions were categorized by education, experience, and job scope.

In-house program staff received higher salaries in every position category. The widest range in salaries was seen at the upper level jobs: regional operations manager, health promotion director, and other top operations jobs.

Although compensation is not the only factor in staff retention, it is a primary consideration for professionals in the industry. By being included in the corporate compensation structure, health promotion staff will have the opportunity to participate in corporate benefits, bonuses, and internal job opportunities.

The primary concern about in-house programs is the cost. With higher staff salaries and benefits, the cost for staffing an in-house program can be considerably higher than using an outside vendor. This additional cost must be weighed against the benefits of staff retention, strategic continuity, and ease of integrating the health promotion program with other business units. One way to assist in program integration and staffing is to create an in-house health promotion committee composed of volunteers representing the various departments within the organization. Their charge is to assist in coordinating health promotion program design, implementation, and evaluation to help other employees reach their health goals.

Outsourced Programs

A variety of factors have contributed to a shift away from health promotion programs being provided solely by in-house practitioners to services being at least partially (if not solely) delivered by management firms and outside vendors. A dramatic increase in employment costs often makes companies concerned about adding to the head count in the form of full-time or part-time health promotion staff. Furthermore, the changing role of health promotion in managed care, the need for more broad-based service delivery models, and the need to serve more geographically dispersed employees, sometimes require specialized products and services to be delivered by outside providers with greater resources. Outside specialists often can provide best-practice services with greater efficiency. There are many important considerations in selecting outside vendors. See appendix 1 for a checklist for making effective selections.

SUMMARY

By understanding the "customer," knowing the resources available, and selecting the appropriate management approach, the best operating plan for the health promotion program can be selected. As previously stated, there is no one correct approach, but the plan must meet the specific needs of the organization. The plan must also remain flexible so that it can evolve as the organization and its needs evolve.

REFERENCES

Association for Worksite Health Promotion. 1997. *Worksite health professionals national compensation survey*. New Brunswick, NJ: Johnson & Johnson Health Care Systems, Inc.

Elliott, S. 1998. *Health and productivity management consortium benchmarking study*. Ann Arbor, MI: American Productivity and Quality Center and the Medstat Group.

Harris, J.H., J.F. McKenzie, and W.B. Zuti. 2002. Anybody out there? *Absolute Advantage* 1(4):4-5.

Chapter 5

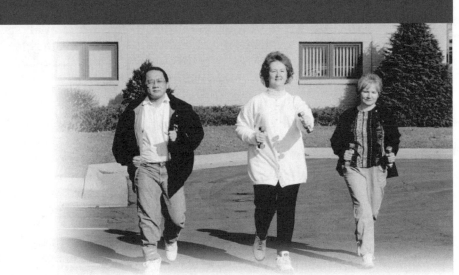

Designing Health Promotion Programs

The health promotion programs that are best practices (those using innovative, imaginative ideas with the potential to improve business results) are systematically planned and comprehensive in nature. Successful programs blend a wide range of program offerings with cultural and environmental support to make the greatest impact and include four important cornerstones:

1. Needs assessment and evaluation
2. Effective interventions
3. Relapse prevention
4. Healthy culture development

All of these cornerstones or components are interrelated. For instance, needs assessment and evaluation directly determine what intervention programs are needed and identify what can be done to develop a healthy culture. In turn, the results of these activities are assessed through needs assessment and evaluation. Likewise, relapse prevention and its success helps determine appropriate interventions and must be supported by a healthy culture. Each of the four cornerstones has a relationship to the others, either supporting them, being supported by them, or both.

NEEDS ASSESSMENT AND EVALUATION

A number of avenues are available for the health promotion program planner to obtain needs assessment and evaluation data. Some data are available directly through health promotion program initiatives such as health-risk appraisals or employee interest surveys. Other data must be obtained through collaboration with human resources, benefits, occupational health, or workers' compensation departments within the organization. Further, some data, while not a direct measure of a company's specific employee population, can be obtained through various county, state, and federal health agencies.

Needs assessment and evaluation are interdependent. Evaluation is performed to assess needs. As needs are understood and then addressed through interventions, reevaluation occurs to determine the outcome of the intervention and to shed light on new needs or changes in approaches required to better meet the original needs.

NEEDS ASSESSMENT AND EVALUATION APPROACHES

Systematic evaluation should be conducted to determine health promotion program needs and to assess the progress of any ongoing activities toward achieving the mission and meeting the established goals and objectives. Evaluation involves initial and periodic needs analysis and quality review as well as the longitudinal assessment of program results across time. The information obtained from evaluation

45

can be used to establish the program design, improve it, or to optimize the desired outcomes and to provide data to justify sustaining the program and enhancing its growth and evolution.

As with most data-oriented processes, the computer and its software are paramount in data collection and in the evaluation of health promotion programs. With the advent of widely available and easy-to-use database software, collection and storage of data have become routine. However, decisions must still be made on what to collect and how to collect it.

While a number of software packages are available to collect fitness center data, few exist that are packaged specifically for other types of health promotion programs. As a result, health promotion professionals are often left with creating their own software with assistance from the internal information services department or by using the system of an external vendor. There are even some organizations that specialize in warehousing data and in external data measurement and evaluation.

Specialty Software Packages

Some specialty software packages available perform the following functions:

¬ Forecast the return on investment of health promotion programs, including both medical and productivity costs

¬ Take health risk appraisal or various types of psychographic data, and cross-analyze it to identify areas where programs are needed and persons who could benefit from different types of programs

¬ Take insurance data and identify modifiable claims opportunities

¬ Survey or audit information on attitudes, culture, and health beliefs

¬ Provide statistical analysis of data collected

TYPES OF NEEDS ASSESSMENTS AND EVALUATION

Needs analysis determines the needs and interests of the people and organization being served. This information can then be used in selecting programs, within the constraints of budget.

Program evaluation usually involves the assessment of process, impact, and outcomes. Additionally, value analysis is often conducted to determine the overall value of the program, taking a number of factors into consideration.

¬ Value analysis determines which program offerings produce the greatest benefit for the lowest cost. A relative value can than be established for each program. This information can be used in selecting future programs, within the constraints of budget.

¬ Process evaluation analyzes the qualitative aspects of program delivery, such as enrollment, participant satisfaction, and effect of mode of delivery on participation. Periodic quality assurance checks related to providers, equipment, and program operation and delivery should also be included in the process evaluation.

¬ Impact evaluation assesses the immediate behavioral, attitudinal, knowledge, and cultural changes that occur as a result of the program. Examples include lifestyle behavior changes, level-of-readiness for behavior change, and changes in health beliefs.

¬ Outcome evaluation determines the success of the program in affecting health-related outcomes such as health status indexes, morbidity, or mortality. It can also be used to examine the program's effect on economic outcomes such as productivity, absenteeism, workers compensation claims, and health care utilization. Economic outcome evaluation often involves cost-effectiveness, or the unit cost of providing a service or of achieving a specific health outcome; cost savings, or the actual reduction in the cost of medical care; and cost-benefit ratio, in which the savings from a program are compared with the cost of providing the program.

NEEDS ASSESSMENT AND EVALUATION DESIGN

In performing an evaluation, an appropriate design must be selected on the basis of what is being assessed. In designing the appropriate evaluation process, consider the following factors as well as those in appendix 2

¬ Data sample. What sample of the employee population should be used to obtain the data? In many cases, the entire population is utilized. However, for sake of simplicity, sometimes a smaller sample may be chosen.

¬ Data collection. How should the data be collected? Data collection can be time consuming, tedious, and costly. However, if not collected, data and thus valuable information are lost forever. Data can be collected via paper, computer, or telephone, but eventually they must reside in a computer database. Once collected, they can then be manipulated and studied.

¬ Data analysis techniques. What techniques should be used to analyze the data? Strengths and weaknesses of the evaluation design, as well as factors affecting the validity of the results, must be addressed in making data analysis design decisions. Issues such as the difficulty of ongoing longitudinal analysis, transience of the population, and the cost of maintaining the data analysis effort must be considered.

¬ (I) Data integration. The data required for analysis are often outside the control of many health promotion professionals. As a result, cooperation must be received from various areas within the organization. Assuming cooperation and commitment are received, data from multiple sources must be integrated for evaluation. Once data are integrated, health promotion professionals should report information valuable to each department involved as well as report information valuable to the overall organization.

NEEDS ASSESSMENT TOOLS

To perform a comprehensive needs assessment, attempt to collect data from as many of the following sources as possible: health risk assessment, biometric screening, employee interest survey, management assessment and corporate culture audit, claims analysis, and indirect sources.

Health-Risk Assessment

Health-risk assessment (HRA) is generally accepted as a central component of an effective health promotion program. HRA serves the dual purpose of creating individual assessment and motivation for behavior change as well as providing valuable group planning and evaluation information. HRA should not be seen as a stand-alone intervention. It is most effective when closely tied to a wide range of educational and supportive interventions.

Caution: Many health promotion practitioners have made the mistake of investing too much of their resources in HRA. While HRA is a very important component, without the necessary resources for diligent follow-up, program success will not be achieved. HRA alone will not create behavior change.

HRA Types

HRAs come in a variety of types and price ranges. HRAs can be found in self-scoring formats, computer-scannable questionnaire forms with extensive result booklets, phone-based tools, and interactive on-line versions. The type of HRA selected will depend on the demographics of the population, program budget, and program data needs (i.e., evaluation or targeted intervention). See the Society of Prospective Medicine's (1999) suggestions for choosing an HRA instrument presented in appendix 3.

Additionally, it is essential that HRAs be conducted in a confidential manner. If HRA results are to be used for individual targeted interventions or incentive programs, consent must be obtained from participants. This requirement may necessitate using a third-party vendor to conduct the HRA to ensure employee confidentiality. Employees need to know that company personnel will not have access to their personal health information. By providing a strong sense of confidentiality, a company can ensure that participation will be greater and participants will be more open and honest in their responses.

Biometric Screening

Many health promotion planners combine HRA with biometric screenings. This technique not only serves as a draw for program participation but also adds a direct-measure component to the program's planning and evaluation efforts. Selection of the screening measures varies from organization to organization. One set of guidelines often used by experienced professionals is the recommendations of the United States Preventive Services Task Force (USPSTF) (United States Preventive Services Task Force 1996). These guidelines are both research based and comprehensive. See table 5.01 for the most common screening measures. Also see appendix 4 for other sources of screening standards and recommendations.

It is important to understand that not all organizations, including the American Cancer Society and various health insurance groups, agree with the recommendations of the USPSTF. Each health promotion staff will need to explore the recommendations and select screening components best suited to their own philosophies and those of their organization and health insurance provider.

Interest Survey

Another valuable needs assessment and evaluation tool is the interest survey. The interest survey can often be combined with HRA and screening programs. The purpose of the interest survey is to focus on the topics and program formats most attractive to employees. Although many HRA tools include some surveys of interest, they are not usually very extensive and generally require supplementation. Interest surveys often include

¬ risk reduction program interest (cholesterol, blood pressure, nutrition, and physical activity);

¬ risk reduction readiness levels;

¬ life-enrichment program interest (life balance, financial health, personal growth, and parenting);

¬ physical activity interests (walking, running, or aerobics);

¬ program format preferences (seminar, class, computer, or self-help);

¬ program time preferences (before work, lunch, or after work);

¬ self-care interests (consumerism issues, headaches, and child illnesses);

¬ preferred communication channels; and

¬ willingness to be involved (wellness committees, support group leader, or physical activity club leader).

Management Assessment and Culture Audits

Longitudinal studies often demonstrate that a majority of lifestyle-change attempts are unsuccessful in an unsupportive environment. Cultural norms and values are effective predictors of both who attempts and fails health-related change and who succeeds (Garner and Wooley 1991). Products and services now exist that can assess the level of support in the organization for maintaining good health and recommend appropriate improvements. In auditing the culture, variables to consider include norms, values, coworker support, organizational support, and work climate. Understanding the environment or culture of the organization is important in determining its overall needs. The level of support can be measured, improved, and engineered to provide the most supportive environment possible.

Additional Sources of Planning Information

Numerous additional sources of planning information data are available to the persistent health promotion planner. Not all of this information is easy to obtain. However, a growing number of health promotion professionals are using this information to better integrate their programs with the other health management efforts within the organization being served.

A short summary of these data sources follows:

¬ Health care claims. Health care claims can provide important insights into the health needs of the population. Working closely with the benefits and human resources departments will be required to access these data. Analysis tools are available to review claims data for self-care priorities, disease management, high-risk areas, and lifestyle-improvement opportunities.

¬ Employee assistance programs (EAPs). All employee assistance programs provide periodic reports of program utilization. This information can provide data about those problems that most frequently trouble employees. The need for topics such as stress management, financial health, parenting, and depression is often identified in this way.

¬ Workers' compensation. Workers' compensation data can identify injury patterns. Working with the occupational health or medical departments can lead to collaborative solutions through programmatic or environmental initiatives.

Table 5.01

The Most Common Screening Measures and Health-Risk Assessment

BIOMETRIC	TEST PERFORMED	PURPOSE	RECOMMENDATION
Total cholesterol	Finger-prick or veni-puncture; fasting not required for screening purposes	Heart disease risk factor awareness	Highly recommended
HDL cholesterol	Finger-prick or veni-puncture; fasting not required for screening purposes	Heart disease risk factor awareness	Highly recommended
Glucose	Finger-prick or veni-puncture; fasting not required for screening purposes	Diabetes risk factor awareness	Highly recommended for at-risk individuals
Blood pressure	Performed either manually or electronically	Heart disease risk factor and stroke risk factor awareness	Highly recommended
Body composition	Skinfold, infrared, or electrical impedance methods	Assessment of obesity, a heart disease and diabetes risk factor	Growing concern over the value of body fat testing. Does it help with weight loss efforts or encourage diet cycling?
Flexibility	Sit-and-reach and back extension tests	General fitness and injury prevention awareness	Recommended where injury prevention is a high priority
Strength	Push-ups, curl-ups, and bench press	General fitness and injury prevention awareness	Recommended where injury prevention is a high priority
Cardiovascular fitness	Submaximal bike or treadmill tests most common; some direct-measure VO_2 testing is occurring at the worksite	Cardiovascular fitness level, a heart disease risk factor	Recommended, but for individual assessment and prescription, not for mass screening purposes
Mammography	Mobile mammography, (not always available) provider partnership is possible	Early detection of breast cancer	Recommended where available (insurance provider partnership is possible)

¬ Short-term and long-term disability. The causes and costs associated with disability are another important source of general health promotion services. Local professionals such as doctors, nurses, and dietitians will sometimes provide services for managing these illnesses.

Indirect Sources

In some cases, obtaining needs assessment and evaluation information for a population is not possible, cannot be obtained for a certain behavior or condition, or a company may choose not to use limited resources on assessment and evaluation. Looking for locally available data sources is prudent when it is likely that the company's health statistics are similar to the local population. Several indirect sources, such as federal, state, and county agencies, are available and can provide useful information in program planning.

R One such source is the Behavioral Risk Factor Surveillance Survey. This program, sponsored by the Centers for Disease Control and Prevention and administered through state health departments, provides prevalence information about a variety of health behaviors for all 50 states. Goals on prevention may be obtained through Healthy People 2010, which is administered by the United States Department of Health and Human Services, Public Health Service. Other voluntary health agencies such as the American Heart Association, National Safety Council, American Lung Association, and the American Cancer Society may be able to provide additional prevalence information. Colleges and universities in the region can also be a useful source of health-planning information.

EFFECTIVE INTERVENTIONS

Over the past 10 years, interventions have increased in sophistication and effectiveness. Most experienced health promotion program planners recommend offering a balance between population-based initiatives (physical activity campaigns, nutrition education, self-care, and stress management) and targeted interventions for individuals who have high risk factors for disease (tobacco use, high cholesterol, high blood pressure, and diabetes). In this way, persons with special health concerns obtain the individual assistance they need, while efforts are made to keep the remainder of the population at lower risk levels.

AWARENESS STRATEGIES

R Some of the most creative ideas in worksite health promotion are used to generate awareness. As a general rule, awareness programs are not intended to create behavior change. Instead, they serve to encourage both readiness for more extensive programs and to remind participants of certain health behaviors. Awareness programs are especially effective in moving contemplators to a preparation or action stage. See table 5.02 for examples of awareness strategies.

EDUCATIONAL STRATEGIES

As suggested earlier, health promotion experts agree that the provision of a variety of health education communications and educational programs is critical for program success for two reasons.

First, not all employees are ready for behavior change in a particular health-risk area at the same time. If one chooses to offer only a single intervention, such as a multiple-session smoking-cessation course, the program would not reach those individuals who are not yet ready to participate. As a result, multiple points of entry, at different times throughout the year, are required.

A second reason a variety of options are needed is that not all employees prefer to learn in the same way. Some individuals choose to learn through group programs, others elect to use self-help materials, some like the flexibility of phone-based programs, and others prefer the computer for obtaining the health information they need.

R The number of educational tools available to the health promotion practitioner has grown dramatically over the past few years. Previously, multiple-session classes were the predominate method of behavior change programs. Increasing demands on employee time, a better understanding of the differences in learning preferences, more outcomes data on what works, and the use of the readiness-to-change model have compelled health promotion planners to offer a wider range of program options. Examples of common educational strategies are presented in table 5.03.

Table 5.02

Awareness Strategies

STRATEGIES	EXAMPLES
Posters	Promote the importance of bike helmets through posters on bulletin boards.
Brochures	Create self-care awareness by placing brochures of the most common everyday illnesses (such as colds, flus, fevers, and back pain) in brochure racks in high-traffic areas.
Displays	Encourage winter activity by placing a display featuring cold-weather exercise apparel at building entrances.
Newsletters	Employee health newsletters create awareness on a variety of topics and also often reach the family.
Bulletin boards	Foster awareness of low-fat fast-food options by having a quiz on low-fat versus high-fat choices.
E-mail messages	Encourage breast health awareness through an e-mail postcard to all women over age 50 during breast health month.
Web page	Seasonal or monthly awareness messages can be placed on the health promotion program home page. Links can also be made to other service agencies with similar messages.
Special events	A group walk on National Employee Health and Fitness Day creates awareness of physical activity.

POPULATION-BASED PROGRAMS

Population-based health promotion efforts are those programs designed to maintain the majority of employees at low risk. Population-based programs have evolved in three categories: risk reduction, medical self-care and consumerism, and life enrichment. This section explores common topics and interventions in each area.

Risk Reduction

Risk-factor reduction programs continue to be a central focus of worksite health promotion. Research has demonstrated the risk factors that are significant health care cost drivers for most organizations (Goetzel et al. 1998). However, initiatives to foster lasting risk-factor reduction in these different areas have had mixed results.

Nutrition Initiative
¬ Include both the topics of low-fat eating as well as weight management.

¬ Address efforts to combat societal messages that portray unrealistic body weights.
¬ Encourage healthy body image.
¬ Promote balanced eating and regular physical activity.
¬ Utilize an intense approach. Research shows that the effectiveness of nutrition education programs increases with the level of program intensity.

Physical Activity Initiative
¬ Provide facilities such as on-site fitness centers to facilitate easy access to physical activity for many employees.
¬ Provide space for on-site aerobics classes.
¬ Provide walking and running paths and shower facilities.
¬ Provide individual consultation with an exercise physiologist or other health professional to assist employees in planning

Table 5.03

Common Educational Strategies

STRATEGIES	DESCRIPTION
Seminars	Topics such as stress management are presented in seminar format.
Classes	Multiple session classes remain a strategy used in tobacco cessation, low back education, weight management, and other complex behavior change areas.
Phone-based	A relatively recent strategy, phone-based programs have been used in tobacco cessation, stress management, nutrition education, and disease management.
Computer-based	Intranet- or Internet-based and CD-ROM–based programs are becoming more common.
Self-help materials	Self-help behavior change programs on a variety of health-risk areas are available from a number of different vendors, usually combining written materials with audiotapes.
Individual consultation	It is becoming increasingly more prevalent to have health professionals such as dietitians, exercise physiologists, and health educators meet periodically with employees on an individual basis.

safe and lasting physical activity programs.

Stress Management Initiative

¬ Focus efforts on both physical and psychological health.

¬ Address cultural and managerial issues.

¬ Involve departments such as training and development or employee assistance in addressing cultural and managerial issues.

¬ Consider management and leadership training, time management, workspace redesign, increased organizational communication, flexible schedules, and telecommuting as part of the stress management effort.

¬ Utilize a holistic approach to stress management by exploring topics such as life balance, self-esteem, and volunteerism.

¬ Utilize a combination of group programs, self-help programs, and phone-based initiatives.

¬ Utilize nicotine replacement therapies.

¬ Utilize a variety of media, including video, audio, computer, and telephone.

¬ Recognize the psychological and chemical addictive components of tobacco use in cessation efforts.

¬ Address worksite smoking policy and smoke-free environments.

Back Care and Injury Prevention Initiative

¬ Utilize a comprehensive approach.

¬ Include on-site analysis of job stations and biomechanics.

¬ Include management training.

¬ Include employee educational programs.

¬ Include ergonomic interventions.

¬ Include ongoing education and reminder systems.

¬ Consider on-site rehabilitation centers.

Medical Self-Care and Consumerism

Helping employees gain the ability to make informed decisions about their health care and interact with the health care system has become a growing responsibility of comprehensive health promotion programs. Further, compared with other health promotion programs, self-care can have an impact in a short period of time (1 to 2 years).

P Some specific medical self-care recommendations include the following:

¬ Utilize a self-care resource book and or self-care nurse lines.

¬ Consider the use of computer-based CD-ROM or contracted intranet or Internet self-care tools.

¬ Provide communications designed to periodically remind employees of the self-care resources available to them. These communications can include newsletter articles, educational displays on seasonal self-care topics, self-care trivia raffles, and brochures on common self-care topics.

Health Care Consumerism

Health care consumerism focuses on the employee's interaction with the health care system. A better understanding of how to interact with the system enhances care and treatment efficacy. Issues to be addressed in health care consumerism education programs often include

¬ choosing a physician;

¬ understanding the role of the primary care physician;

¬ making the most of office visits;

¬ talking with the physician;

¬ managing prescription and over-the-counter medications; and

¬ making decisions about surgery.

Preventive Services

Compliance with recommended preventive examination schedules continues to be surprisingly low. Provide programs that

¬ create awareness of the examinations recommended;

¬ inform when it is time to begin each type of preventive examination;

¬ inform on how often preventive examinations should be scheduled;

¬ provide information on the importance and value of each preventive examination;

¬ address both child and adult immunizations;

¬ utilize awareness education materials such as posters and pay envelope stuffers;

¬ utilize computerized reminder systems to send paper or electronic reminders to targeted populations using age and gender parameters; and

¬ deliver on-site screenings when practical and appropriate.

Life Enrichment

In the past decade, health promotion programs have expanded greatly in the area of life enrichment. Understanding that optimal health is more than just limiting physical health-risk factors, many health promotion professionals have begun to address such topics as:

¬ work and family balance;

¬ parenting;

¬ grandparenting;

¬ emotional intelligence;

¬ financial health;

¬ elder care;

¬ communication;

¬ self-esteem;

¬ body image;

¬ volunteerism;

¬ complementary medicine; and

¬ living wills.

While these topics are generally presented in seminar formats, other methods and locations have included

¬ resource centers;

¬ resource phone lines;

¬ resource fairs; and

¬ on-site demonstrations.

TARGETED HEALTH INTERVENTIONS

Over the past 10 years, health promotion has become progressively more focused on the specific needs of the individual. These targeted interventions have been particularly applied to participants who have been identified as being at higher risk or who are already diseased. Whereas this approach is sometimes more expensive on a per-participant basis, it is often more cost-efficient because it focuses on only those services necessary or specific to the identified needs of the participant.

Targeting Case Study

The following case study illustrates the value of targeting. One morning at a general practitioner's office, 10 patients arrive over the course of the first hour, all complaining of a sore throat. The receptionist directs them all into a large examining room as they arrive. By the end of the hour, they are all assembled and sitting together. The doctor walks in and, only confirming that they all have sore throats, prescribes the same drug for all of them. Unfortunately, as health promotion professionals, we know that some could have a viral sore throat that would receive little value from medication. Others might have a bacterial sore throat that would respond to antibiotics. Yet, others might have simply screamed too loud at the basketball game the night before or, at the other extreme, might have a throat tumor. The point is that individuals have different health promotion needs and thus need targeted programs.

Targeting has advanced well beyond making sure that the correct content is provided to an individual on the basis of risk or disease. Factors being considered in targeting include risks, diseases, learning style, level of support, readiness for change, desired location of contact (home or work), and a variety of other factors. The descriptions of the targeted health interventions that follow provide additional information on state-of-the-art approaches.

Disease Management

Over the past several years, both health promotion professionals and the medical establishment have embraced the concept of disease management. Disease management is an outgrowth of medical case management that focuses on impacting specific chronic diseases. Although still evolving, effective disease-management programs focus on both the clinical and the behavioral aspects of any given chronic disease. They also identify candidates by the level of morbidity and cost identified through medical and pharmaceutical claims analysis.

To provide services most cost-efficiently, diseases are often classified by level of acuteness, with persons whose diseases are most acute treated more aggressively than persons whose diseases are less acute. The primary functions of disease-management programs are to maximize the well-being of the chronically ill employee or dependent and to minimize the cost generated by repeated hospital admissions, emergency room treatments, and other potentially avoidable medical expenditures.

Diabetes Disease–Management Case Study

The patient has a history of diabetes, chronic lung disease, and cardiomyopathy. Diabetes had been diagnosed several years previously, but the patient had never received diabetic education. In addition to the previously diagnosed illnesses, the patient was recently found to have urinary incontinence and benign prostate hyperplasia.

The preintervention treatment plan was follow-up with an endocrinologist for the diabetes.

The disease-management intervention was as follows:

- A relationship was established between the disease-management RN counselor and the patient.
- Ongoing follow-up with the counselor continually provided the most appropriate medical care.
- A formal outpatient diabetic education program was instituted.
- A special consultation was received from an endocrinologist.
- Ongoing telephone counseling support for behavioral issues, including weight loss, better nutrition, and self-care, was established.

Outcome

Diabetes management resulted in the patient's blood sugar returning to average. The patient now monitors blood sugar four times a day and better manages lifestyle-related factors.

Prognosis

While this patient's history does not lead to a good prognosis, it is anticipated that the appropriate management of the diabetes will minimize the number of acute-care stays in the hospital and improve or maintain quality of life.

Employee Assistance Programs

Employee assistance programs (EAPs) have been in existence for many years and have stood the test of time. EAPs provide employees and their dependents expedient access to help for a variety of types of personal problems, by phone or in person. This help is provided with maximum confidentiality, given that it is delivered outside of the normal health care coverage. The primary purpose is to intervene with assistance before the personal problem escalates or, if it has already escalated, to accelerate the participant's referral to the appropriate type of care.

EAPs are commonly used with employees who have substance abuse; alcohol misuse; and marital, mental health, financial, or other personal problems. EAPs also often provide educational programs for supervisors to help them recognize problems and other initiatives that have a positive impact on the mental health of the population, while controlling mental health and productivity costs.

Kellogg Company Case Study

The Kellogg Company offered an exemplary managed mental health initiative, part of which includes EAP services provided to over 6,000 employees based in the United States. Although EAP utilization rates generally fell within optimal limits, the Kellogg Company recognized that utilization rates alone were not a true measure of effectiveness. The company continued to work toward a goal of analyzing how effectively the EAP met established goals and objectives, continually refining the program to improve outcomes. The program was integrated within a strategic plan addressing a full spectrum of mental health needs, including assessment, education, intervention, and short-term and long-term treatment (see figure 5.01).

United Auto Workers and General Motors Corporation Case Study

In 1996, the United Auto Workers (UAW) and General Motors Corporation jointly sponsored the Lifestyle Management (LM) pilot program, an intervention designed to provide individualized advising to persons identified as high risk as part of its comprehensive LifeSteps health promotion program. The objective of LM was to facilitate long-term behavior change among workers, retirees, and their spouses. By taking into consideration demographic, geographic, psychographic, and health metric factors, LM facilitated follow-through, provided motivation, and targeted preventive efforts toward the risk area(s) of each individual. Additionally, the participant's LM advisor provided on-going monitoring and guidance to keep the individual directed toward reducing risk factors.

The UAW-General Motors Corporation Lifestyle Management Program

To most effectively control both the impairment and the cost of work-related injury or illness, both preventive and proactive disability management strategies must be adopted. These initiatives must be targeted to the unique personal and job-related needs of each individual. Targeted strategies used in the occupational health setting include safety and other injury prevention strategies, functional capacity testing, ergonomics, physical and occupational therapy, and worker readiness.

Safety and Other Injury Prevention Strategies

Individuals should be targeted with specific safety and other injury prevention strategies on the basis of their specific job types. For instance, stretching exercises specific to a given job (designated by job number) can be provided to workers, with various incentives to perform the exercises as a preventive measure.

Functional Capacity Testing

Functional capacity testing is often used to proactively assess an employee's ability to perform work before or after injury and is usually used under three circumstances:

1. To determine a potential employee's capacity to perform a given job before placement

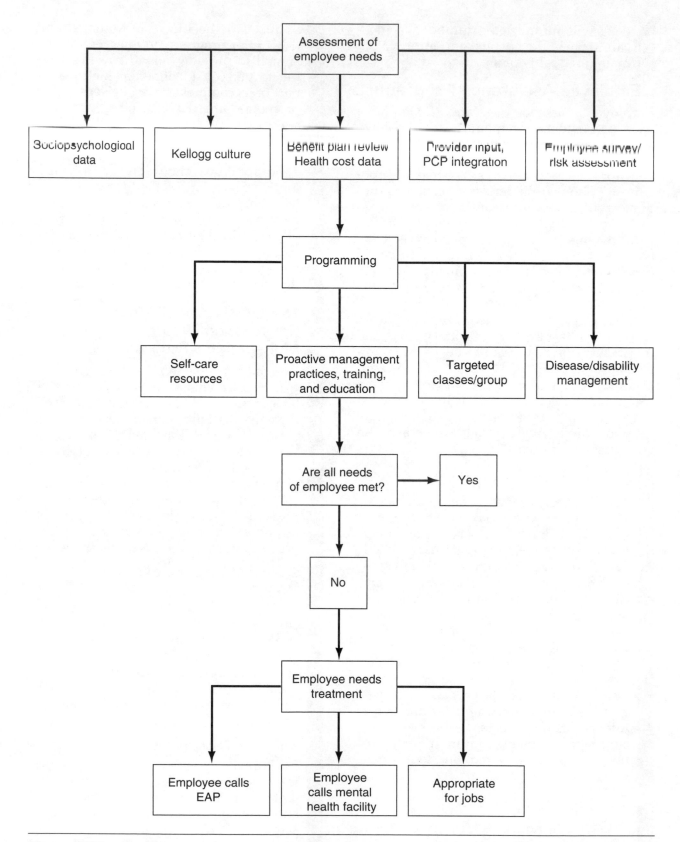

Figure 5.01 Employee needs assessment flow chart.

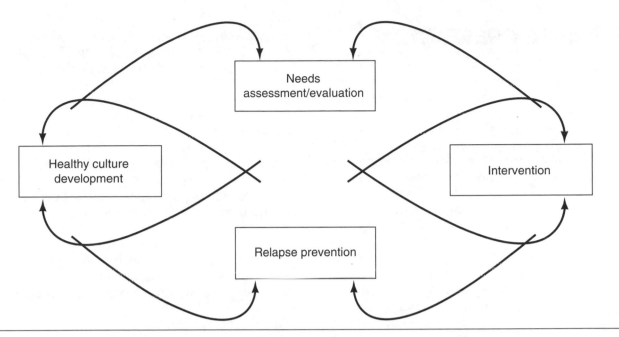

Figure 5.02 Needs assessment flow circle.

2. To periodically test employees' abilities to perform their jobs as factors change (age, new equipment, or a change in the way the job is performed)

3. To determine if an injured worker has the functional capacity to perform the job without risk of reinjury

Functional capacity testing ensures that the worker's functional capacity is adequate to perform the job assigned without risk of injury to the worker or others.

Ergonomic Programs

In a working environment, there are job tasks that can contribute to injuries such as sprains and strains. Targeted ergonomic programs can be developed to identify the jobs on which injuries commonly occur and to make workstation design changes that will reduce the incidence of injury.

Physical and Occupational Therapy

When a worker is injured, targeted physical and occupational therapy should be used to expedite return to work at a functional capacity necessary to safely perform the assigned job. To accomplish this objective, the following types of targeted rehabilitation are often used.

¬ Passive modalities are used primarily during the acute injury phase to reduce symptoms affecting the individual's ability to perform and tolerate therapeutic exercise. Very few industrial rehabilitation conditions require a reliance on passive modalities.

¬ Therapeutic exercises are used to proactively restore the muscular range, strength, endurance, power, balance, and coordination necessary to meet the physical job demands.

Worker Readiness

Worker readiness programs provide targeted activities to make certain that workers are physically and mentally prepared for work after healing and rehabilitation of primary injuries. Worker readiness usually involves a full-body exercise program, balance development, agility work, aerobic training, and general conditioning. Additionally, measures are implemented to assist the employee in coping with the psychological and social aspects of the injury. Health promotion programs are used to address any dietary, stress, or other lifestyle factors that could contribute to reinjury. Worker readiness programs targeting the injured employee help ensure that overall functional capacity is adequate to perform the assigned jobs at the earliest possible time.

RELAPSE PREVENTION

Relapse prevention addresses the greatest challenge facing health promotion programs, the maintenance of positive health behavior changes. Maintaining behavior change through relapse prevention strategies is critical, if the program is to result in improved productivity, reduction of health risk, and management of health-related costs.

Relapse prevention continues to be the greatest challenge to worksite health promotion programs. While short-term behavior change successes are commonplace, long-term maintenance of these changes has not been as successful. The most important strategy in relapse prevention is the continuation of the comprehensive mix of programs over time. Searching for and implementing new and creative ways to address long-standing health behavior problems such as inactivity and poor eating habits is one of the best defenses against relapse. Following are three strategies commonly used to prevent relapse.

SUPPORT GROUPS

Support groups have been offered in worksite settings for some time with mixed results. The ongoing maintenance of the groups is usually the biggest barrier. Strong peer leadership and periodic educational events can help to keep support groups viable.

REMINDER SYSTEMS

Many health behaviors, such as compliance with preventive screening examinations, can be maintained through systematic reminder systems. Reminder postcards or e-mail messages distributed on specific occasions (i.e., birthdays, holidays, or national observances) have proved to be very effective. Further, reminder systems such as memos, brochures, and newsletters have been used to continually encourage individuals working to reduce blood pressure, cholesterol levels, or other physiological parameters to persevere.

INCENTIVES

Another growing, yet relatively unproved, method of providing ongoing support for behavior change is incentive-based programs. Incentives designed to encourage year-round participation in health promotion programs have been successful in increasing participation. Incentives can be financial awards, gifts, or other tangible rewards. There is some concern about the extrinsic nature of incentives and the difficulty for individuals to internalize health improvement efforts when incentives are involved (Robison 1998). However, there seems to be some evidence that extrinsic rewards can create motivation until such times that intrinsic reward is realized.

Incentives have been used since the earliest health promotion programs. They were first used in the promotion of physical activity. Mileage clubs, where participants earned prizes for accumulating exercise mileage, were common. In the past decade, many health promotion practitioners have continued to utilize incentives as a part of their health promotion programs. However, the types and scope of the incentive programs have grown significantly. Following are examples of incentive programs and a chart describing typical incentive awards.

Participation-Based Incentives

The most common form of incentive programs are participation-based incentives. With this type of program, employees are rewarded for their efforts to participate in health promotion programs regardless of individual outcomes. Typical participation categories used include

¬ physical activity efforts;

¬ compliance with recommended preventive service examinations;

¬ participation in self-care and health care consumerism programs;

¬ participation in health-risk reduction programs; and

¬ participation in life-enrichment programs.

Risk-Rated Insurance

This type of incentive program utilizes health assessments and screenings to identify and reward those employees determined to be at low risk. For example, if a person were to have a cholesterol level of 150 mg/dl, he or she would be eligible for the reward, whereas a person with the cholesterol level of 250 mg/dl would not. The Health Insurance Portability Act has made the provision of differential benefits based on health-risk status illegal, and thus new variations of this concept that work within the law are being utilized by some organizations.

Gain Sharing

This form of incentive program is based on rewarding all employees when the health care expenditures for the organization are less than expected in any given year. A percentage of the difference between expected and actual health care expenditures is divided between the company and the employees.

TYPICAL INCENTIVE AWARDS

Typical incentive awards usually include cash, flexible benefits, merchandise, and time off.

Cash Awards

Cash awards ranging from $50 to over $1,000 have been used. Savings bonds are another popular choice. The tax implications of cash awards must be taken into consideration. Also, considering that a year is a long time to wait for an award, quarterly or more periodic awards are sometimes used.

Flexible Benefits

Additional flexible benefit dollars have been made available by some companies to reward employees for health promotion efforts. This type of award necessitates coordination of a number of logistical considerations with the benefits department.

Merchandise

Employees in this type of award system earn points or "well bucks" to purchase a variety of merchandise. The merchandise usually is health and fitness related, such as walking shoes and exercise apparel.

Time Off

While not often used, time off from work can be an effective incentive for health promotion activity.

HEALTHY CULTURE DEVELOPMENT

Healthy culture development can support health promotion efforts, increasing the potential for success. Although changing culture is a long-term process, appropriate support enhances employee readiness for behavior change and creates an environment in which it is both acceptable and encouraged. Awareness programs, statements from senior leadership, health-friendly company policies, and financial support for the health promotion program are all helpful in creating a healthy culture.

A healthy culture is a process that involves the development of openness, trust, belief in people, relationships, learning, achievement, business performance, and confidence. Although the process is time consuming and requires firm commitment from both management and employees, the value it brings to the well-being of the organization is well substantiated. Traditionally, these efforts to improve the work culture have been called organizational development and have focused on human interaction as it relates to accomplishing work.

Table 5.04 illustrates strategies and examples of what can be done to create a healthy environment within an organization.

Table 5.04

Strategies for a Healthy Organizational Environment

STRATEGIES	EXAMPLES
Facilities and stress	Showers, walking and running paths, fitness centers, relaxation relief rooms, access to health-related Web sites
Food service	Salad bars, low-fat selections, fresh fruit vending, farmers market, labeling programs
Policies	Tobacco policies, seat belt policies, safety policies
Benefits strategies	Preventive service coverage, incentive programs, flexible work hours, flexible benefits to include health improvement
Management training	Leadership, communication, and stress management

In a healthy worksite environment, not only are the human interactions positive and productive but also policies, practices, resources, and support make adhering to good health habits more easily accomplished. To build a healthy environment, support is needed from leadership, and cooperation is required throughout the organization. The health promotion professional can be the catalyst for changes that can help build a healthy environment. Often the changes required are small, but when combined, they can create an environment that is collectively conducive to maintaining a healthy lifestyle.

A healthy worksite, combined with a healthy environment, can create a culture that is maximally conducive to health promotion. The more visible the support mechanisms, the more likely employees will view healthy lifestyle as an acceptable or even expected norm within the culture.

SUMMARY

Planning health promotion programs around the four cornerstones of needs assessment and evaluation, interventions, relapse prevention, and healthy culture development will generate the best possible results. These components allow the program to determine need; encourage, educate, and support positive health behavior changes; and support those changes with the widest possible audience.

REFERENCES

Garner, D., and S. Wooley. 1991. Confronting the failure of behavioral and dietary treatments for obesity. *Clinical Psychology Review* 11:729-780.

Goetzel, R., W. Anderson, W. Whitmer, R. Ozminkowski, R. Dunn, J. Wasserman, and the Health Enhancement Research Organization Research Committee. 1998. The relationship between modifiable health risks and health care expenditures: An analysis of the multi-employer HERO health risks and costs database. *Journal of Occupational and Environmental Medicine* 40:843-854.

Robison, J. 1998. To reward . . . or not to reward? Questioning the wisdom of using external reinforcement in health promotion programs. *American Journal of Health Promotion*. 13:1-3.

Society of Prospective Medicine. 1999. *SPM handbook of health assessment tools*. Pittsburgh, PA: The Society of Prospective Medicine: Institute for Health and Productivity Management.

United States Preventive Services Task Force. 1996. *Guide to preventive services, 2nd edition*. Baltimore: Williams & Wilkins.

Chapter 6

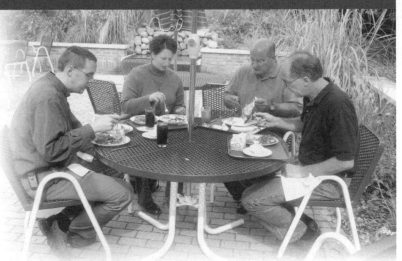

Using Administrative Processes and Procedures

The four cornerstones of health promotion programs—needs assessment and evaluation, effective intervention, relapse prevention, and healthy culture development—cannot exist without sound administrative procedures and people who will develop and implement those procedures. The administrative processes are the mortar that not only holds the cornerstones of a health promotion program together but also links and binds the program to overall organizational goals.

The Association for Worksite Health Promotion (AWHP) Board of Directors appointed a Professional Standards Task Force to develop professional guidelines for worksite health promotion directors (HPDs). The task force developed 96 competencies for the position that have been validated and published (Association for Worksite Health Promotion 1995). The main functions of the HPD are divided into three broad areas: (1) human resource management, (2) business management, and (3) program management.

The HPD must develop and implement sound policies and procedures within each of these areas to operate a successful health promotion program. A best-practice health promotion program must have sound administrative systems and procedures in each of the core areas. These administrative systems and practices must be interrelated and linked to organizational policies and procedures and must be consistent with industry standards.

AREA 1: HUMAN RESOURCE MANAGEMENT

Perhaps most critical to the overall operation of a worksite health promotion program is the process of attracting, hiring, and training key personnel. What staff positions are necessary and how will those positions be filled? Who will run the program and what are the duties, responsibilities, and necessary credentials for each position?

Many organizations have developed certification programs for health and fitness professionals. The American College of Sports Medicine (ACSM) offers different levels of certification within two specific tracks: (1) health and fitness and (2) clinical. The health and fitness track includes certifications for exercise leader, health and fitness instructor, and health and fitness director. These certifications are appropriate if you are working with exercise participants who are apparently healthy or have controlled diseases and are exercising for health maintenance.

The clinical track includes certifications for exercise specialist and program director. These certifications are designed for individuals who work in clinical settings where participants will, in most cases, be at increased risk for exercise-related events (American College of Sports Medicine 1999). While many other certifying organizations exist, the ACSM is recognized as a leading certifying body within the industry. The knowledge, skills, and abilities included in the ACSM certification include the following:

¬ Functional anatomy and biomechanics

¬ Exercise physiology

¬ Human development and aging

¬ Pathophysiology and risk factors

¬ Human behavior and psychology

¬ Health appraisal and fitness testing

¬ Emergency procedures and safety

¬ Exercise programs

¬ Nutrition and weight management

¬ Health promotion

Another certification available for health promotion professionals is the certified health education specialist (CHES). CHES certification covers the following areas of responsibility for entry-level health educators (National Commission for Health Education Credentialing 1994):

¬ Assessing individual and community needs for health education

¬ Planning effective health education programs

¬ Implementing health education programs

¬ Evaluating effectiveness of health education programs

¬ Coordinating health education services

¬ Acting as a resource person in health education

¬ Communicating health and health education needs, concerns, and resources

STAFFING THE HEALTH PROMOTION PROGRAM

A number of preliminary considerations must be taken into account before the hiring process is initiated. Determining staffing needs on the basis of the health promotion program plan is the first step in this process. This determination can be made by a wellness team or the organizational component or representative who will oversee the health promotion program. Staffing levels and job descriptions will depend on the scope of programs and services offered, number and type of eligible participants, budget parameters, internal and ex-

ternal resources available, and desired outcomes. Once staffing needs have been determined and approved, the staffing process includes

¬ conducting a job audit;

¬ developing a task analysis;

¬ writing job descriptions;

¬ developing performance standards and qualifications;

¬ finding candidates for the jobs;

¬ interviewing and evaluating job candidates;

¬ contacting references;

¬ hiring top candidates;

¬ orienting new employees to their jobs, the program, and the organization; and

¬ managing staff changes using proper legal and organizational policies and procedures.

RECRUITING AND INTERVIEWING

Many sources are available from which to recruit qualified employees, including Internet job sites, professional magazines and journals, newspapers, colleges and universities, personal health promotion networks, employment agencies, and industry-specific search firms and professional associations. In many organizations, internal job postings occur before external efforts are initiated. The health and fitness industry, like others today, struggles with attracting and retaining high-quality employees.

The STAR (situation, task, action, results) method is an efficient process that focuses on past behaviors to predict future behaviors. This method helps by investigating recent, relevant, and future trends. Candidates are asked to respond to interview questions by giving specific examples in which a situation developed or a task was assigned, outlining the action that was taken, and finally explaining the results of that action. See appendix 5 for STAR interview questions and guidelines.

The interview process requires skillful execution, considerable time, and experience on the part of the interviewer to obtain the best available candidate for the position. The candidate should be interviewed by the person to whom he or she will report and by the human resources department if one exists. Once the core competencies have been discussed, the interview questions should follow a specific pattern to focus on results.

Some important legal issues must be considered when conducting job interviews and hiring employees. Your organization should have a written policy governing hiring procedures. Following are some basic hiring guidelines and considerations:

¬ When checking references, stick to facts. You can acquire more than just a confirmation of dates of employment as long as the information is factual and documented in the personnel file. This information could include a job description, salary range, and a stated reason for leaving if the employee provides one. Ask for permission to acquire this information.

¬ You cannot ask a potential employee about past injuries, but you can ask the candidate if he or she has any present conditions that might limit or restrict his or her job performance.

¬ Do not raise the issue of children. Simply inform the candidate of the required hours including any overtime that might be required.

¬ Gender only becomes a qualification for positions when work tasks could be compromising (such as a locker room attendant). Gender balance can be a long-term goal but should not be an issue with a specific position.

¬ Personal grooming is a legitimate hiring consideration; however, you should avoid height and weight issues and not make them factors in the hiring process.

¬ If an employee's religion forbids work on any particular day, an employer is required to accommodate that worker's religious needs unless such measures would create an undue hardship on the business. Courts seldom recognize "undue hardship," so it is best to offer accommodations when possible. Many options are available, such as swapping shifts, making up hours, or using flexible schedules.

¬ Know and understand the Americans with Disabilities Act (ADA) as it relates to hiring and firing. For example, drug abuse is a recognized medical condition covered by ADA. However, the ADA excludes current illegal drug use from protection. Alcohol abuse is protected even if an employee is still drinking. Usually, employers accommodate substance abuse by giving employees time off for treatment. Some ongoing psychological conditions are also covered under ADA if they meet certain requirements.

¬ Sexual harassment is defined by the Equal Employment Opportunity Commission as unwelcome sexual advances, requests for sexual favors, and other verbal or physical conduct of a sexual nature. The definition covers practices ranging from direct requests for sexual favors to workplace conditions that create a hostile environment for males or females. Sexual harassment is not about sex; it is about power and the abuse of power.

JOB DESCRIPTION

S ≡P Typically, job descriptions are partially dictated by the specific environment and needs of an organization. A comprehensive set of job description characteristics include

¬ date;

¬ title of position;

¬ division or department;

¬ who is writing the description;

¬ supervisor;

¬ location of position;

¬ exempt or nonexempt from overtime pay;

¬ overview (summary) of expectations of the job, principal accountabilities (often assigned a percentage value), and job activities;

¬ kind and level of internal and external contacts required of this position;

¬ decisions made and acted on independently;

¬ decisions referred to supervisor for appraisal or final disposition;

¬ duties with respect to employee development, placement, work assignments, and salary administration if any;

¬ number of full-time equivalents reporting to this position, budgetary and organizational responsibilities, and characteristics of the department that add complexity or difficulty to job performance;

¬ minimum qualifications and skills;

¬ personal characteristics (self-motivation, communication, interpersonal skills); and

¬ physical demands (equipment, machinery, ability to lift a specific weight, work in extreme temperatures).

In worksite health promotion, job classifications vary greatly according to the size of the facility operation (if appropriate), scope of services offered, location of programs to be delivered, and number of participants.

Generally, the health promotion program director is ultimately responsible for all aspects of program development, budgeting, capital development, marketing implementation, and evaluation. Larger programs may have an assistant program director position. In both positions, it is highly desirable to have ACSM program director's certification or the ability to apply for and complete this certification within an allotted period of time.

The health educator or health promotion specialist is responsible for planning, coordinating, and delivering the various programs. In many facility-based programs, staff are cross-trained to handle multiple activities in both fitness and exercise prescription, as well as health education programs. Although there is no clear standard for the ratio of professional staff to participants in non–facility-based health promotion programs, it is generally accepted that a maximum ratio of 1:200 (staff to participant) is appropriate in a full-service facility-based model.

TRAINING AND DEVELOPMENT

Once a candidate is hired, the most crucial period of employment begins. Realistic expectations should be communicated clearly to new hires along with a thorough introduction to the company's culture, team environment, and all human resource processes. Probationary periods, lasting from 30 to 180 days, give the employee and the employer an opportunity to see if there is a good "fit" for long-term employment. During this period, employment can be terminated at will under most employment arrangements.

The human resources department usually handles inducting new employees into the company. Every new employee should receive an employee handbook outlining

¬ company history, philosophy, and mission;

¬ organizational chart;

¬ employment classifications;

¬ employment policies;

¬ standards of conduct;

¬ performance and compensation;

¬ benefits;

¬ leave;

¬ insurance coverage; and

¬ training and education.

In developing staff, it is necessary to create a challenging and motivating environment. The right combination of flexibility, freedom, and professional growth is essential to building a winning team.

INDEPENDENT CONTRACTOR

An independent contractor provides specific services to an organization on a contract basis. The use of independent contractors in the health and fitness industry has become increasingly popular for a variety of reasons. An organization using an independent contractor is not required to pay FICA (Federal Insurance Contributions Act, or Social Security), FUTA (federal unemployment), or state unemployment taxes. In addition, the independent contractor does not receive employee benefits. With the steady increase in employee benefits and other employee costs, this arrangement may be perceived as a real benefit to employers.

The independent contractor and the contracting organization must consider several legal issues before classifying someone as an independent contractor. If ignored, these issues expose the business, and possibly the contractor, to financial and, perhaps, serious legal consequences.

20 Factor Test

The Internal Revenue Service (IRS) applies a ruling known as the "20 Factor Test" to determine if workers are employees or independent contractors. A "yes" answer to any of the questions would indicate that the person is an employee and not an independent contractor. An employment lawyer can help classify people appropriately. Appendix 6 shows the 20 Factor Test.

Typically, independent contractors are not covered under an organization's general liability insurance policy. An organization should require all independent contractors to carry liability insurance, show proof of coverage in the form of a current certificate of insurance, and make sure that the organization is listed as an additional insured on the policy.

AREA 2: BUSINESS MANAGEMENT

In this era of megamergers, acquisitions, and alliances, businesses are constantly changing. Business cultures are forced to change overnight in the wake of mergers or corporate restructuring. Experience indicates that even a best-practice health promotion program can be cut or eliminated during these dynamic times. The profound changes taking place in the workplace illustrate the importance of aligning health promotion program goals with the business's priorities and understanding the relationship between the two.

Although business management skills may seem out of the realm of interest and expertise of the health promotion professional, they are a prerequisite for becoming a health promotion director. There are eight areas within business management that define expectations for the health promotion director:

¬ Technological applications
¬ Facility and equipment
¬ Financial management
¬ Organizational policies and procedures
¬ Communications
¬ Marketing
¬ Business planning
¬ Quality management and assurance

TECHNOLOGICAL APPLICATIONS

To be technologically competent, the health promotion professional should be able to select appropriate software and other technologies for the health promotion program. Software needs differ greatly for a facility-based program that will require membership tracking and, possibly, billing and cash collection. Suggested system features to consider for a facility-based program include

¬ master database;
¬ form letters;
¬ membership renewal process;
¬ merchandise sales;
¬ locker rental fees;
¬ financial statements;
¬ reports;
¬ purchase order system;
¬ petty cash system;
¬ bank statement reconciliation;
¬ basic inventory management;
¬ member check-in;
¬ fitness assessment and exercise program;
¬ health-risk assessment; and
¬ member goals and activity tracking.

The health promotion director must also be able to identify organization and management data needs and integrate technological applications of the health promotion program into the worksite environment.

FACILITY AND EQUIPMENT

Management of a health promotion program includes the ability to provide facility design, equipment recommendations, and space layout plans. For a program that includes a fitness center, the selection of exercise equipment requires specific consideration of function, cost, space, durability, safety, versatility, user appeal, and maintenance.

To be competent in equipment and facility management, the health promotion director must be able to identify appropriate equipment and space needs; develop a system for inventory control; develop an equipment and facility maintenance schedule; and identify any environmental, structural, and legal design issues that will affect the health promotion program delivery. Appendix 7 provides a sample checklist for exercise equipment maintenance and cleaning.

FINANCIAL MANAGEMENT

Whether operating in a corporate, community, hospital, or other setting, health fitness managers must be familiar with standard financial principles and procedures to compete in today's marketplace. To be competent in the area of financial management, the health promotion director must be able to develop an operating and capital budget for the health promotion program, present and defend the budget, interpret financial statements, and manage the budget effectively (see table 6.01).

Good financial management begins and ends with a planning process that links outcomes to program goals. The numbers are only as good as the plan that goes with them. The budget provides the road map that leads to the achievement of the program goals. A worksite health promotion budget will consist of the expected income (if any) from the program and anticipated expenses for a specific time. Revenues received in a health promotion program are often not large, if they exist at all, but do require a process by which they are accounted. Fees for screenings, copayments for classes, and fitness center membership fees are examples of income. Budget preparation includes developing an operating budget, a capital expenditure budget, and a cash budget. The budgeting process is a team process and should include team coordinators, supervisors, and managers who are involved with the health promotion program.

¬ The operating budget summarizes the financial projections (income and expenses) for all phases of the health promotion program. The operating budget can be built from previous budgets or from the ground up (zero-based budgeting). Each income and expense category is broken down into line items. The operating budget (and capital budget) should be developed approximately 3 months before the end of the fiscal year.

¬ The capital expense budget determines the future cost projections for the building and equipment. In preparing this budget, the health promotion director must consider replacing assets that may be obsolete, worn out, or inefficient. In addition, new projects and program expansion may necessitate new or additional equipment. The capital budget typically includes any piece of equipment that costs more than $500 with a useful life of at least 1 year.

Capital expenses will be placed on the operating budget as a depreciation expense over the life of the instrument. For example, a $1,000 bicycle ergometer used for exercise testing would be expected to have a working life of at least 5 years. The ergometer would be placed in the operating budget as a depreciation expense of $200 per year ($1,000 divided by 5). It is not uncommon for capital expenses to be on a separate budget time line than the rest of the operating budget.

¬ The cash budget provides a period-by-period estimate of the amount and timing of cash flow. This budget may be broken down into quarters, months, weeks, or a year. This budget reflects the estimated cash inflows and outflows of normal operations. A cash-flow budget encourages management to identify, evaluate, and monitor financial variables that affect the program.

The budget preparation process begins with identifying the overall program goals and creating the action and intervention plans and steps that will lead to goal achievement. The budget process is a continual process that differs from setting to setting; however, there are basic steps that are appropriate in any setting. They include the research phase, goal and objective development, draft development, management review, final budget review, and implementation (see table 6.02 for a sample program budget).

EXPENSE MANAGEMENT

Understanding the expense side of operating a health promotion program is a key component of financial management. Controlling expenses begins with categorizing all costs associated with operating the program. From there, each major expense category can be subdivided into standard industry expense categories. Expenses can be divided into variable expenses and fixed expenses.

¬ Variable expenses are those expenses that vary depending on the level of employee participation. Most of the costs for

Table 6.01

Steps to the Budget Process

STEP	INTERVENTION	ACTION PLANS
Step 1	Call to action	Announce the budget process to all involved, and provide a format and workable timetable for completion. The previous year's results can be distributed if available. Select a method for projecting income and expenses. Use zero-based budgeting (starting from "scratch") or percentage increases (giving each line item a set percentage increase).
Step 2	Research	Review historical financial data and the prior year's budget; look at current year-to-date income statement. Look for trends or variances to help determine patterns.
Step 3	Goal and objective	Determine how the health promotion program will develop and operate in the next fiscal year; include financial goals and assumptions based on overall management profit plan for the organization.
Step 4	Draft development	Draft budget should be as close to the final budget as possible. It should be completed 2 months before the start of the new year.
Step 5	Management team	Share the draft budget with your management team review at least 1 month before the start of the new year. Determine and finalize any changes to the budget. Work for "buy-in" and approval from all involved.
Step 6	Finalize budget	Once the management team signs off on the budget, present to senior management for approval and discuss highlights. Once approved, distribute copies to your team.
Step 7	Implementation	Implementation begins on the first day of the new fiscal year. Review results monthly and compare actual financial results with the budget. If there is a large variance, favorable or unfavorable, budget modifications can or will be made.

program interventions fall into this expense category. To calculate the variable expense needs for the program, participation must be estimated. Participation rates vary by industry, degree of promotion, and maturity of program. Benchmarking of other similar organizations in the area may be necessary to properly estimate participation. Variable expenses include screening, health-risk appraisals, classes, and incentive awards.

¬ Fixed expenses are those that remain fixed or constant for a given period of time. Changes in fixed costs may be expected and do occur over long periods of time. Fixed costs include rent, utilities, salaries, benefits, insurance, and property taxes.

¬ Depreciation is the process of allocating the cost of a long-term asset over its estimated useful life as an expense. Depreciation is listed as a real expense on an income statement. Before depreciation can be determined, you must estimate the asset's useful life and determine its expected salvage value.

Table 6.02

Sample Program Budget

BUDGET ITEM	UNITS	COST PER UNIT ($)	WORKING LIFE (YR)	TOTAL ANNUAL COST
INCOME				
Aerobics copayment	2,880 participants	1.50/participant		$ 4,320
Tobacco cessation copayment	40 participants	25/participant		$ 1,000
CAPITAL EXPENSES				
Desk	2	800 each	5	$ 320
Chair	2	350 each	5	$ 140
Computer	2	4,000 each	5	$ 1,600
Printer	1	1,000 each	5	$ 200
Software	4	150 each	3	$ 200
FIXED EXPENSES				
Staff salaries				$ 70,000
Staff benefits				$ 16,100
Office space	300 ft^2	20/ft^2		$ 6,000
Phone costs	2 phones	720/phone		$ 1,440
Professional membership	AWHP membership	150		$ 150
Professional subscriptions	2 subscriptions			$ 400
Legal fees				$ 500
Employee health newsletter	5,000 employees	2.75/employee		$ 13,750
Office supplies				$ 1,250
Promotional materials				$ 2,000
Educational seminars	16 seminars	200/session		$ 3,200
VARIABLE EXPENSES				
Cholesterol screening	2,500 participants	15/participant		$ 37,500
Blood pressure screening staff	125 staff hours	40/hr		$ 5,000
Health-risk appraisal	2,500 participants	15/participant		$ 37,500
Tobacco cessation program	40 participants	125/participant		$ 5,000
Self-help educational materials	200 booklets	2.50/booklet		$ 500
Aerobics classes	240 hours	22/hr		$ 5,280
Incentive prizes	500 participants	5/participant		$ 2,500
Total income				$ 5,320
Total expenses				$210,530
Total				$205,210

ORGANIZATIONAL POLICIES AND PROCEDURES

(I) Establishing standardized policies and procedures that provide for safe, effective, and consistent administration and operation of a health promotion program is a primary responsibility of the health promotion director. This responsibility includes determining what the policies are; integrating the policies with overall corporate policies; and complying with current professional standards and state, federal, and local laws in all areas of operation.

(R) The American College of Sports Medicine (ACSM) Health/Fitness Facility Standards and Guidelines (2nd edition) is a key resource for health and fitness professionals (American College of Sports Medicine 1997). It provides accepted standards and guidelines by which facilities, staff, and programs can be evaluated. This text is a recommended resource for all facility-based programs. It presents the standards that must be demonstrated by all health and fitness programs and facilities.

The ACSM standards and guidelines book summarizes key findings into six major categories:

¬ Screening of facility members

¬ Supervision of youth services and programs

¬ Demonstration of professional competencies

¬ Utilization of appropriate signage

¬ Emergency response planning

¬ Compliance with laws, regulations, and standards

The text also sets forth guidelines for operating procedures and design features that would enhance the quality of service that a facility provides to its users and provides sample forms to assist the health and fitness professional. Included are sample forms for informed consent, waiver, physician's release, release of information, and emergency procedures, all of which are necessary for facility operations.

LIABILITY AND LEGAL CONSIDERATIONS

Operating a health promotion program, which may or may not include an on-site facility, presents inherent risks for participants and personnel. An environment that may include health screenings, health assessments, group exercise classes, indoor and outdoor recreational equipment and facilities, cardiovascular and strength training equipment, locker rooms with wet areas, and, possibly, whirlpools and swimming pools has the potential for accidents and injuries. An accident or injury could result in a lawsuit against an organization, a vendor, an independent contractor, or an employee. For these reasons, professionals operating health promotion programs must be knowledgeable about and protect themselves from legal issues and liability.

The potential legal consequences of a poorly handled incident in a health promotion setting could be significant. The best line of defense against a serious incident is a well-developed and well-managed risk management program and a competent, well-trained staff.

This section will address some of the legal concerns and responsibilities of nonmedical health professionals. The goal is to identify major areas that could generate legal questions and provide resources and examples to assist the health promotion professional in evaluating and managing risk. The information presented here is not intended as legal advice but rather as guidance. No forms or legal documents or contracts should be adopted by an organization or a program without being reviewed by legal counsel.

The definitions in table 6.03 are important because they determine, in part, when a court might award damages for an injury. In a health fitness setting, the most likely areas for tort liability will be issues of negligence. To substantiate a charge of negligence, the court must prove (1) the existence of a legal duty to protect a person from injury, (2) that there was a breach of that duty, (3) that damages or injury did occur, and (4) the act of the defendant was the proximate cause of the injury.

ON-SITE FITNESS CENTERS

Organizations with on-site fitness centers expose themselves to a higher degree of risk and uncertainty than most businesses with non-facility health promotion programs. The greatest areas of risk for fitness facilities are slip and fall injuries. A 1996 study conducted by Royal Insurance of Charlotte, North Carolina, showed 31% of all claims against fitness facilities were

Table 6.03

Key Areas of Responsibility for Health Promotion Professionals

KEY AREAS	RESPONSIBILITIES
Health screening and assessments	Confidentiality Physician's clearance Waivers and informed consents (see tip box on page 72)
Contracts and agreements	Membership Vendor
Equipment	Maintenance and cleaning Placement Proper usage and supervision
Creating safe environments	Physical plant Signs Security Emergency procedures
Personnel	Qualifications Certifications Employees vs. independent contractors (see box on page 65)
Employee handbook	State and federal laws OSHA ADA Copyright Harassment

for slip and fall injuries. The next largest number of claims (8%) and costs incurred were for injuries sustained while using equipment (Grantham et al. 1998). These statistics highlight the need for special risk management standards and practices when operating fitness centers or recreational programs and activities.

The ACSM standards and guidelines book also provides detailed facility operations guidelines (American College of Sport Medicine 1997).

Detailed equipment maintenance and repair logs should be kept and updated daily or as noted in a facility operations manual. These records may be crucial in the event of an equipment-related incident or injury. See appendix 8 for a sample Fitness Facility Inspection Report form.

INSURANCE

There has been an unprecedented growth in malpractice claims against health care professionals recently. This trend absolutely mandates the need for adequate liability insurance coverage. While health educators and fitness professionals may have once been considered a low-risk group for lawsuits, recent trends demonstrate that even the exercise specialist is not immune from suits and is in need of professional liability insurance.

While proper risk management practices will help reduce the chances of a lawsuit, suits will occur against health promotion programs and professionals. Thus, it is important to understand the types, costs, and availability of insurance needed to protect those who operate health promotion programs. It is also important to know the exclusions included in a policy. Adequate liability insurance coverage will help minimize the financial consequences of a major lawsuit and bring the health promotion professional peace of mind.

Types of insurance to consider include the following:

¬ General liability insurance, which all health and fitness professionals should have or be covered by. This insurance covers claims for bodily injury resulting from general negligence. Read the policy carefully. Know and understand basic content, limits of coverage, and exclusions (e.g., sexually transmitted diseases, martial arts, physicians, physical therapists, and liquor liability).

¬ Professional liability insurance insures professionals against medical claims in negligence suits. Professional liability could be included on a general liability policy or could be added by paying an additional premium.

¬ Personal injury insurance provides protection against suits involving libel and slander.

¬ Property insurance protects against loss of a building and its contents, usually for losses caused by fire, smoke, wind, hail, riot, and vandalism.

¬ Workers' compensation covers the actual medical cost and wages lost for injuries sustained by an employee who is under the supervision of an employer. An employer is required to have this coverage for all employees. Cost is based on the size of the payroll.

¬ Employment practices liability insurance covers employers for liability for employment-related practices. This insurance will extend to claims, charges, and lawsuits alleging discrimination on the basis of age, color, disability, national origin, religion, and sex and also to allegations of sexual harassment and wrongful termination.

¬ Employee dishonesty insurance provides coverage when there is intent by an employee to cause an employer a loss. The loss usually involves cash, but it can also involve taking property or allowing an unauthorized discount on a purchase.

¬ Commercial automobile insurance covers losses for bodily injury or property damage to third parties caused by automobile accidents. Liability can arise from using rented, borrowed, or employee-owned cars that are driven on behalf of the business.

¬ Umbrella liability insurance provides excess coverage over and above that provided by the general liability, auto liability, and employer liability policies. Usually the umbrella policies provide broader coverage than the primary policy. Premiums are not subject to rate regulations.

P To maximize the chances of operating with safety and protection against liability, follow this checklist and the tips in the Tip box on page 72.

¬ Keep program records confidential and stored in a locked file cabinet. Release records only in case of emergency or for legal purposes. **R**

¬ Know and follow the standards of care in the industry as prescribed by the ACSM, the American Council of Exercise (ACE), the American Heart Association (AHA), the National Committee for Quality Assurance (NCQA), and the Occupational Safety and Health Administration (OSHA), as well as all state and federal laws, including the Americans With Disabilities Act (ADA), Equal Employment Opportunity (EEO), and pertinent copyright regulations. See appendix 9 for OSHA excerpt on bloodborne pathogens.

¬ Do not diagnose, treat, or prescribe for any injury or other physical condition, including offering nutritional counseling and dieting advice, unless you have appropriate certification. Do not claim to be something you are not.

¬ Always keep proper documentation. Have a written and up-to-date policy manual, participants' forms, staff appraisals, facility and equipment maintenance records, and all personnel records. Make sure documents are signed and dated whenever possible and appropriate. See appendix 10 for a sample Incident Report and appendix 8 for a Fitness Facility Inspection Report.

¬ Develop and manage a sound risk management plan. Conduct regular safety audits using an in-house team or a third party; ask your insurance carrier if it provides this service.

¬ Review insurance needs carefully and acquire adequate insurance protection for all areas. Require all vendors and other independent contractors to show proof of current insurance, listing your organization as an additional insured.

Contrary to some opinions, waivers are or can be worth the paper they are written on. If they are voluntarily signed by a competent adult; written in clear, readable, and unambiguous language; properly presented; explained to the signer; and comply with state laws, waivers will protect the service provider for injuries resulting from the negligence of the provider. Unfortunately, waiver laws vary considerably from state to state.

A major misconception is that waivers will not protect the service provider if negligence is involved. On the contrary, the waiver is designed to protect the service provider from liability resulting from negligence of the service provider or its employees. However, no forms are effective for gross negligence in which a service provider or employee is consciously indifferent, resulting in an extreme degree of risk.

To be valid, the waiver cannot be against public policy; that is, it cannot be opposed to the best interest of the public. Another requirement for a valid waiver is consideration, or something of value, given in exchange for a promise or for performance.

Waivers continue to protect against lawsuits if they meet proper requirements.

See *The Exercise Standards and Malpractice Reporter*, published by PRC Publishing, Inc., for specific cases involving waivers.

COMMUNICATION

Communication involves the sharing of ideas, information, comments, and complaints among staff, employees, program participants, and management. The success of the health promotion program will depend on effective communication. Knowing what you want to communicate is an important step, but it is only one step in the communication process.

There are different levels of communication needed to develop and sustain a successful health promotion program—from securing senior management support, to identifying and aligning the internal corporate resources, to developing an effective awareness campaign directed at a target audience. Each level of communication has different goals and challenges, but the communication processes are similar. There are basic questions to ask at each stage of the program development process:

¬ What is your purpose for communicating?

¬ Who is your target audience?

¬ What are you trying to communicate?

¬ What resources (financial and other) do you need?

¬ What resources do you have?

¬ What outcome or response are you looking for?

In answering these questions, you can develop your communication how-to plan and identify the steps and methods necessary to achieve your desired results.

COMMUNICATING TO MANAGEMENT

How do you secure senior management support for the health promotion initiative? The first step may be to assess management's readiness to support health promotion and at what level. Behavioral scientist James Prochaska suggests that we may need a model by which to assess decision makers' readiness for change (Prochaska 1997). Prochaska's model recognizes behavior change as a process that unfolds over time and progresses through six stages.

Try to assess where management falls on the readiness scale, and then proceed with some of the following strategies:

¬ What are your competitors doing in the area of health promotion? Distribute competitors' fitness and wellness program materials to senior management.

¬ What are other best-in-class organizations doing? Provide business statistics that show how well "healthy companies" are doing.

¬ What do the employees want? Use an employee survey to create awareness and show interest levels. Provide quantitative and qualitative information. You can use focus groups, employee suggestion boards, and respected employees to champion the cause.

¬ Provide existing research data and statistics to show the beneficial effect of health promotion on employee morale, productivity, absenteeism, medical benefits, and insurance costs.

¬ Link health promotion initiatives to social and community responsibility.

¬ Tie health promotion program to the corporate mission and culture. Challenge the company to prove that employees are its most important assets.

¬ Show connection between reducing health care costs and labor costs; emphasize that health care utilization drives health care costs.

¬ Work with benefits managers to strengthen your case that "good health is good business," and incorporate wellness into the long-term plan for managing health care costs.

¬ Show how program costs can be partially or fully funded through benefits savings such as self-insured health plan cost reductions, higher deductibles, and employee subsidies.

¬ Provide a financial forecast of the potential value of the health promotion program to the organization.

ORGANIZATIONAL COMMUNICATION

While new and existing programs have separate challenges, both require a well-defined, ongoing communication plan that identifies a purpose and a process and provides the tools for successful implementation. Good communication in today's competitive and dynamic business environment means coordinating common functions, reducing or eliminating overlap, and maximizing human and financial resources to create a better organization.

Identifying the infrastructure for communicating to the organization as a whole is a critical step in planning the communication process. Identifying and motivating the appropriate people in the organization and defining their roles in communicating the health promotion message help ensure that the goals will be met. Groups that can be utilized as part of the coordinated effort include occupational health and safety, benefits and human resources, fitness center and recreation, employee assistance programs, unions, and administration.

This integrated approach to health promotion communication is the model being used by most best-practice organizations (see figure 6.01).

Representatives from each business unit and external vendors, when involved, can follow the guidelines listed here in effectively communicating the health promotion program.

¬ Unify the group to a common purpose or vision.

¬ Link program goals to business and health objectives.

¬ Define responsibility areas for all team members.

¬ Identify internal liaison or ownership for each program component.

¬ Establish written, measurable program goals and disseminate to all involved.

¬ Conduct regular meetings (at least monthly) with a clear agenda.

¬ Provide quarterly status updates to senior management and annual updates to employees.

¬ Hold employee focus groups to listen and learn.

STAFF COMMUNICATION

Verbal communication is basic to any business but especially to a service business such as health promotion that relies heavily on personal interaction. We all must communicate, but exactly how clearly, how candidly, and how often depends on the message we are communicating, the audience, the desired results, and the communication style we employ.

Open and effective communication between staff and program participants is critical to the success of a health promotion program. Personal communication provides an immediate opportunity for feedback. Successful communication techniques include

¬ being knowledgeable and believable;

¬ establishing rapport with your audience;

¬ using professional language, not slang;

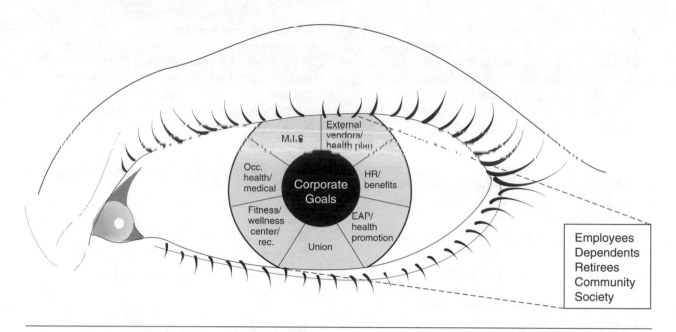

Figure 6.01   Organizational communication: An integrated and focused approach.

¬ speaking in friendly, reassuring, and confident tones;

¬ watching your audience for nonverbal feedback;

¬ listening attentively;

¬ maintaining eye contact;

¬ using open body language;

¬ avoiding jargon, technical terms, abbreviations, and acronyms unless you know your audience understands them;

¬ keeping your message simple and to the point;

¬ being enthusiastic and dynamic;

¬ involving your audience; and

¬ dressing appropriately.

In an environment with open and direct communication, employees know their responsibilities, what is expected of them, and how they stand with coworkers and supervisors. The following are steps suggested by Robert H. Rosen, author of *The Healthy Company*, to communicate effectively in the workplace (Rosen 1991):

¬ Open your eyes and ears: praise, listen, and ask.

¬ Say directly what you want and mean.

¬ Provide sincere, honest, and constant feedback.

¬ Tame office conflict.

¬ More (communication) is better and much more is best.

¬ Don't criticize or reprimand in public.

As in any business environment, conflicts will arise among professionals in a health promotion setting. The current work environment is extremely stressful for many with threats of downsizing, outsourcing, mergers and acquisitions, and the day-to-day challenges of balancing work and family life. Expectations are high, and people are looking for quick answers, quick fixes, and quick results. The health promotion professional must be prepared to face and resolve conflicts.

Conflicts

Here are some steps to follow when conflicts arise:

¬ Defuse the discontent.

¬ Work to agree on the problem.

¬ Research and gather all facts.

¬ Come up with a solution.

¬ Inform all staff of any policy changes.

¬ Follow up with a personal note or call.

When a conflict arises, review the situation with all staff and talk about how the situation was handled. Discuss what was done and what could have been done to resolve the situation and reduce the anxiety level for all. Try role-playing with your staff to prepare them for a conflict before it happens.

COMMUNICATION FOR DIVERSE POPULATIONS

A major challenge facing worksite health promotion professionals is communicating with diverse employee populations. Understanding the various dimensions of diversity is the first step in developing appropriate and meaningful educational materials and media. These dimensions include age, race and ethnicity, family background, educational levels, gender, language, occupation, religion, level of acculturation, and access to resources. Access to resources is a particularly important issue because resources are increasingly becoming accessible only through online communication.

When assessing and reviewing health promotion materials for distribution, health promotion professionals must consider organizational demographics, education and literacy levels, health beliefs and practices, and language capabilities before materials are developed and disseminated.

Certain music, phrases, words, or activities can be very offensive to certain racial, cultural, or ethnic groups, so the health promotion staff must be cognizant of these issues before developing, advertising, and distributing any health promotion materials (Ramirez 1995).

COMMUNICATION TOOLS

Nonpersonal communication, including printed materials, electronic messages, and displays such as bulletin boards and posters, are still necessary to promote and advertise the overall health promotion program and events. Focus groups and special events, such as health fairs, open houses, community and charity events, and outdoor recreational and family activities are also effective marketing tools. Defining your objectives helps you determine if the communication is necessary and what type of communication will be most effective.

New technologies have dramatically changed the way health information is communicated. Taking advantage of technology will enhance an organization's and a health professional's ability to market, deliver, and evaluate health promotion programs. Online tools that simplify the way people access and control information are readily available. These communication tools are being used to promote self-responsibility and the creation and use of individually tailored interventions.

As the Internet continues to grow, the ability to efficiently locate factual and meaningful information is the challenge. Knowing how to evaluate the validity of health recommendations and products on the Internet is important.

Web Site Information

The following list provides guidance on what to consider when evaluating or using Web site information:

¬ What is your purpose or goal?

¬ What are the author's credentials?

¬ Is the information current?

¬ Are scientific references cited?

¬ Are you focusing on the content of information or on graphics?

¬ Do you need permission to copy or distribute the information?

Appendix 11 lists some popular Web sites to explore.

Helpful Web Sites - Healthfinder is a free gateway to reliable consumer health and human services information developed by the United States Department of Health and Human Services. Healthfinder links to carefully selected information from U.S. government agencies, major non-profit and private health organizations, state health departments, and universities. It covers more than 1,000 topics and includes many resources in Spanish.

The National Library of Medicine offers an online database that contains almost 10 million references to journal articles in the health sciences. MEDLINE may be researched free by anyone who has access to the Internet. Searchers can use one of two National Library of Medicine search engines: PubMed or Internet Grateful Med. There is also a link to MEDLINE from MEDLINE plus, the National Library of Medicine's new consumer health Web page.

MARKETING

As health promotion becomes more focused on the specific needs of the individual, the methods of marketing should become more directed and focused as well. The day of advertising a health education seminar or screening exclusively by posting and distributing fliers is gone. While eye-catching, easy-to-read, informative fliers might pique the interest of some, others will need a much more directed approach. The "shot gun" approach to marketing health promotion programs is not a cost-efficient or effective way to get program participation and, more important, to produce health behavior change.

The best way to communicate the health promotion program is to do the following:

¬ Identify the purpose of the program.

¬ Develop the identity, theme, or logo of the program.

¬ Identify and link internal and external resources (i.e., consultants and vendors).

¬ Identify target groups (i.e., employees, dependents, retirees, the community, or high-risk individuals).

¬ Send an introductory letter from the company leadership announcing the rollout of the program.

¬ Notify employees about program goals and specifics.

¬ Communicate incentives for participation (financial or otherwise if they are part of the program).

¬ Hold special events initially and annually to create enthusiasm and momentum for the program (e.g., open house, health fair, or family activity).

¬ Disseminate information in formats appropriate to the audience.

BUSINESS PLANNING

The planning process involves developing a focused mission statement with supportive goals and objectives that complement and support the overall organizational mission and strategies. The business plan provides the road map to effectively manage the short-term and long-term operation of the health promotion program.

The overall guide to a program's direction and resulting successes is the strategic plan. It can be defined as a pattern in a stream of decisions or actions. More than what a business intends or plans to do, the strategic plan is also what the business actually does. The ultimate purpose is to help organizations and business units increase performance through improved effectiveness, efficiency, and flexibility.

Although there is no set format for creating a strategic plan, this working document will address mission and goals, external operating environment, internal analysis, and strategic choice as follows:

¬ Mission and goals are clearly stated definitions of the business you are in that answer the questions of who is being satisfied (customer groups), what is being satisfied (customers' needs), and how customers are being satisfied (by what technologies). These statements also identify the time frame to achieve set goals and how the business will carry them out.

¬ An analysis of the external operating environment identifies strategic opportunities and threats specific to health promotion, the competitive position of any rivals, the stage of the industry's development, and the wider macroenvironment, including social, governmental, legal, and technical issues such as the effect of managed care and population health management on your business.

¬ Internal analysis pinpoints the strengths and weaknesses of your business while identifying the quality and quantity of resources available.

¬ Strategic choice generates a series of alternatives following directly from an analysis of the business's external and internal environment. A SWOT (strengths, weaknesses, opportunities, and threats) analysis assists in matching strengths to environmental opportunities to gain and sustain a competitive advantage.

QUALITY ASSURANCE

"A never ending cycle of continuous improvement . . . is perhaps a fitting definition for continuous quality improvement in the new millennium" (Deming 1982). Similar to the value discipline that shapes an overall strategy, managing and improving quality is the way to continued business success. Centered around a few basic principles—customer satisfaction, continuous improvement, and teamwork—quality is not about changing the way people think about themselves or their jobs but about how people and their jobs work together. It is about facilitating the easiest, most efficient, and most logical flow of materials, ideas, or information between two or more people who together form a process. It is understanding who the customers are, what their requirements are, and meeting or exceeding those requirements without error and on time.

A simple process of continuous quality assurance is to *plan*, *do*, *check*, and *act*. The *plan* focuses on a selected product or service in which customers and their requirements are identified and work processes are rehearsed, understood, and analyzed to identify needed changes. *Do* puts change in motion, while *check* evaluates the effectiveness of the change. Finally, *act* standardizes, communicates and implements the improvements.

W. Edwards Deming, an innovator in quality measurement who revolutionized management philosophy in America during the 1980s, developed 14 points on quality improvement (Deming 1982). These 14 points have become standard in U.S. companies:

1. Plan for the future.
2. Realize the need for change.
3. Strive to eliminate the need to calm dissatisfied customers.
4. End lowest-tender contracts.
5. Improve every process.
6. Institute on-the-job training.
7. Institute leadership.
8. Drive out fear.
9. Break down barriers.
10. Eliminate slogans.
11. Eliminate arbitrary numerical targets.
12. Push pride on the job.
13. Encourage education.
14. Move top management to action.

AWHP's Guidelines for Employee Health Promotion Program suggests 10 quality standards for successful programs (Baun, Horton, and Storlie 1992). Note the similarities to the Deming model. Accordingly, a program must

1. have senior management commitment;
2. form a clear statement of philosophy, purpose, and goals;
3. possess an assessment process for organizational and individual need, risk, and costs;
4. have professional leadership;
5. address significant health risks of the nation, employees, and organization;
6. motivate for lasting behavior change;
7. have effective marketing drives and consistent participation rates;
8. develop efficient systems for program operations and administration;
9. implement evaluation procedures for quality and outcomes; and
10. possess an effective communication system.

REPORTING

In any business, budgets, forecast reports, and strategic plans guide senior managers in making intelligent decisions concerning the overall direction of the company. As a business, health promotion can be measured at select set points over time, and, if needed, corrective measures can be taken to keep the business on track. Business planning is a necessary part of fitness and health promotion programs and is critical to the ongoing success or continuance of the operation.

Monthly operations reports provide a quick reference check on progress and may include

¬ number of participants;
¬ number of programs offered;
¬ utilization rates;
¬ synergies with other departments;
¬ summary of activities;
¬ number of staff and staff-to-participant ratio;
¬ number of accidents and how they were handled;
¬ number of complaints and how they were handled;
¬ number of compliments; and
¬ referrals.

Quarterly reports often offer more insight into cost and health issues and may address topics such as risk status change, health-risk prevalence, changes in claims status and claims utilization rates, and continuous quality initiatives employed in addition to a summary of monthly operations.

The annual report is prepared for senior management and provides valuable information for decision making. It offers a year in review by highlighting key accomplishments and provides quantifiable data, including financial summaries. In health promotion, it should be used to inform others of the benefits of the program and offer an opportunity to showcase the efforts of the program.

Key elements of an annual report include a business component, a program component, and an evaluation component.

Business Component

¬ executive summary (one-page summary recapping highlights of the annual report);

¬ mission statement (how the health promotion division supports the mission of the company);

¬ goals and objectives;

¬ staffing (table of organization and staff biographies); and

¬ financials (income, expense, any cost-saving measures utilized).

Program Component

¬ description of programs offered and accompanying numbers;

¬ description of marketing strategies to implement programs;

¬ what needs to be offered in the future; and

¬ what (other) changes must be made.

Evaluation Component

¬ compilation of objective data of the year;

¬ numbers of participants who started and who completed programs;

¬ utilization;

¬ participant satisfaction (survey results);

¬ participant gender distribution;

¬ participation by topic; and

¬ changes to health status (blood pressure, cholesterol, weight loss or percent body fat loss, impact of behavior).

The annual report is a must for a long-lasting program as it regularly communicates to decision makers the accomplishments and benefits of your health promotion effort.

CRITICAL SUCCESS FACTORS FOR HEALTH PROMOTION EXCELLENCE

Much has been written about the administrative processes germane to successful worksite health promotion programs. Whether ensuring program growth, program continuance, or the possibility of launching a new business opportunity, there are key critical success factors (CSFs) in the areas of business management, program management, and human resource management that need consideration regardless of how your program's success will be measured.

The following CSFs are common threads seen in most best-practice health promotion programs:

1. Management Leadership and Vision Compatibility. The successful worksite health promotion leader will recognize the need to enhance the company's overall mission and vision in all he or she does—in communication with other company leaders through reports, collateral materials, products, and services developed; in communication with vendors and clients; and, perhaps most important, in communication with every participant involved in the health promotion program. Find and share examples of how your work in health promotion furthers the mission, vision, and values of the company you work for. Keep senior leaders routinely apprised of your efforts.

In general, practice what you preach. If you preach teamwork, do you work well with others? If you ask your people to take risks, does your behavior match your words? If you recommend lifelong learning, do you keep current and contribute to this field? Appendix 12 offers insight into effective leadership practices.

2. Accountability and Outcomes. Noted quality, productivity, and management authority, W. Edwards Deming has long been considered the expert in statistical process controls. Yet many of his methods apply to the health promotion industry. One underlying theme in his work is accountability.

As a health promotion leader, you are accountable for results. As a leader, you must delegate responsibility and authority, but you cannot delegate accountability. This level of accountability is best exemplified by delivering appropriate outcomes. Deming refers to five key words when describing outcomes: *what gets measured gets done.*

Clearly, the efforts of your department should produce tangible results. However, for optimal effectiveness, the results must be measurable. Larry S. Chapman, MPH, suggests that some of these measurable outcomes might include

- the accomplishment of formal objectives;
- participation;
- participation feedback (both quantifiable and anecdotal);
- health-risk prevalence change;
- risk status change;
- changes in the stages of readiness;
- utilization and cost effects; and
- cost and benefits and net present value.

3. Operations. The book, *ACSM Health & Fitness Facility Standards and Guidelines* (American College of Sports Medicine 1997), summarizes key operations findings into six major categories.

- Screening of facility members
- Supervision of youth services and programs
- Demonstration of professional competencies
- Utilization of appropriate signage
- Emergency response planning
- Compliance

4. Change Management. We still do not know what direction national or state health care reform will take. However, if economic incentives for demand management initiatives continue, there will be a number of provider demand management strategies that will be utilized. Wellness and health promotion programs will present opportunities to both catalyze and guide the evolution of health care and integrate these changes into the effort to achieve an overall improvement in public health status.

In this age of consolidations, mergers, acquisitions, and reengineering of companies' missions and visions, change is inevitable. Adapting to change will be the key to health promotion program success and, ultimately, to program survival. You must be flexible. At times, there may be a need to take one step backward to move two steps forward.

Changes in Management Structure

Consider the following when faced with changes in management structure or direction:

- Know your position, your mission, and how they relate to the new directions.
- Increase synergy with other departments.
- Link your program to the company's mission, vision, and values.
- Investigate communication styles.
- Learn who has the power to legitimize change.
- Keep key people informed; keep them involved.
- Increase name recognition and visibility.
- Let administrators know they have ownership.

---

5. Information, Documentation, and Reporting. Have clear policies and procedures in place. Make sure the proper authorities (i.e., legal department and human resources) have had an opportunity to review documents. Keep records that report trends over time. Prepare a comparative analysis on what your competitors are doing. Compare data to benchmark standards. Communicate information concisely and in a timely manner to upper management.

Perhaps one of the biggest reasons for nonsupportive management is employees asking for more without justification. Lack of participation, stagnation, low utilization rates, unjustified complaints, and inappropriate referrals all contribute to creating barriers to further support. Conversely, backing requests with proper information contributes to survival.

6. Hire the Best. A health promotion motto includes *people, place,* and *programs.* Of these, it's the people who make the place and programs successful. The STAR approach helps identify the best candidate for the program and the position. Make a new

hire's first assignment as important as anything else he or she will do on the job. Create a sense of ownership among the results they produce.

Nothing is more important to the continuing success of your program than the contributions and commitments your employees make. Hiring the best can ensure the continuity of your program, but keeping them challenged is an art. The proper combination of freedom, flexibility, and professional growth championed by effective managerial leadership will keep your staff challenged.

7. Continuous Quality Improvement. Continuous quality improvement is a process of monitoring and measuring performance against established quality standards to consistently improve a product or service.

If you don't involve yourself with the continuous quality improvement process, you won't have to worry about customer satisfaction. Someone else will satisfy your customers for you.

You sustain a competitive advantage in business by being the best, not necessarily by being the cheapest. To be the best, you must take your customers seriously and give them what they need, not what you think they need. In a competitive world, health promotion will succeed if there are guarantees of quality in the goods and services delivered.

8. Resource Integration. Do not forget about opportunities to cross-market services within your organization. This effort will further your position within your company as a division that is well connected and an integral part in the success of other departments.

9. Responsiveness. Empower your frontline staff to resolve customer issues on the spot and provide continuous training for those who make the first impression on customers. You never get a second chance to make a first impression.

10. Financial Management and General Business Savvy. Treat all cost centers as profit centers. One of the knocks on health promotion programs, especially in not-for-profit companies, is that they do not always operate like a true business. Understand

the difference between mission and margin. Remain sensitive to other cost centers in your company. Even though labor as a percentage of expenses is steadily increasing, consider contracting for services or utilize part-time staff (less than 20 hours a week), when appropriate. Employ other economies of scale and cost efficiencies whenever you can, and be sure upper management is aware of your efforts.

The following outlines business savvy needed by new entrants to the field as well as by seasoned veterans:

Professionals Entering the Field

¬ Sharpen writing, speaking, and reading skills.

¬ Develop a results-oriented mentality; focus on outcomes.

¬ Remember that special populations need attention. Often 5% of a company's workforce is responsible for 65% of their health care costs.

¬ Figure out how you will add value and then demonstrate it.

¬ Ask yourself four questions every day: What am I doing? What should I be doing? What should I not be doing? What should I be doing next?

¬ Know the issues facing community health improvement.

¬ Understand operating (financially) as a mission versus margin.

¬ Become familiar with relationship marketing.

Experienced Professionals

¬ Read all you can on financial measurements and ratios, budget processes, technology interventions, marketing, and health care issues.

¬ Align with physician health improvement efforts.

¬ Know the CSF of your department.

¬ Speak the language of finance.

¬ Develop a profit center mentality.

¬ Apply activity-based costing strategies where appropriate.

¬ Understand managed care, population health management, and other industry terms and their impact.

¬ Know issues facing physicians as gatekeepers.

¬ Anticipate regulatory and legal requirements.

¬ Be intimately familiar with and implement continuous quality improvement initiatives.

¬ Benchmark best practices (appendix 13 highlights key management and employee relations practices of the Fortune 100 Best Companies).

Proper business conduct is the responsibility of every new and experienced employee. Although it is difficult at times to differentiate between ethical and legal issues that arise, most companies will have policies dealing with key issues as they relate to the law. However, if you are in doubt about any situation, it's always best to *stop*, *think*, and then *act*. Ask yourself the following questions:

¬ Is it legal?

¬ Does it follow company policies and value structure?

¬ Is it ethical?

¬ How will it look in the newspaper?

¬ Can the decision be defended to others?

¬ Am I treating others the way I want to be treated?

¬ Is it in the best interest of the customer?

SUMMARY

Even with all the best intentions, efforts, planning, and preparation, some programs may not survive changes in senior leadership or a shift in core strategies. What preparations are you working on to thwart efforts to limit or cut your program? Every business has a strategy. Make what you do at the health promotion level lead to a sustainable competitive advantage for your company.

REFERENCES

American College of Sports Medicine. 1997. *Health/fitness facility standards and guidelines, 2nd edition*. Champaign, IL: Human Kinetics.

American College of Sports Medicine. 1999. *ACSM Certification Resource Catalogue*. Champaign, IL: Human Kinetics.

Association for Worksite Health Promotion. 1995. How do you measure up?—Guidelines for the worksite health promotion director. *Worksite Health*. Fall: 18-23.

Baun, W.B., W.I. Horton, and J. Storlie. 1992. *Guidelines for employee health promotion programs*. Association for Worksite Health Promotion. Champaign, IL: Human Kinetics.

Deming, W.E. 1982. *Quality, productivity, and competitive position*. Cambridge, MA: Massachusetts Institute of Technology Center for Advanced Engineering Study.

Grantham, W.C., R.W. Patton, T.D.York, and M.L. Winick. 1998. *Health fitness management*. Champaign, IL: Human Kinetics.

National Commission for Health Education Credentialing. 1994. Renewals and certification handbook for health education specialists. Allentown, PA: National Commission for Health Education Credentialing, Inc.

Prochaska, J. 1997. Understanding the changes of change paradigm. *Worksite Health* Spring: 8-12.

Ramirez, S. 1995. Health communication: Developing educational materials and media programs for diverse employees. *Worksite Health* Winter: 13.

Rosen, R.H. 1991. *The healthy company*. Los Angeles, CA: Jeremy P. Tarcher, Inc.

Part II Summary

The operating plan may be the single most important element of a successful health promotion program. Programs range from being delivered primarily in-house to being delivered primarily by external providers. Health promotion programs can be successful regardless of where they fall on this continuum, but when planning the program, a decision must be made as to how the program will be operated. Often this decision will be based on what you are trying to achieve, the management approach preferable in the corporate culture, and the resources available.

Systematic evaluation should be conducted to determine health promotion program needs and to assess if any ongoing initiatives have been successful in achieving the mission and meeting the goals and objectives established. Evaluation involves initial and periodic needs analysis and quality review as well as the longitudinal assessment of program results across time. Over the past 10 years, interventions have increased in sophistication. Most experienced health promotion program planners recommend offering a balance between population-based initiatives (physical activity campaigns, nutrition education, self-care, and stress management) and targeted interventions for individuals at increased risk for disease (tobacco cessation, high cholesterol, high blood pressure, and diabetes). Relapse prevention addresses the greatest challenge facing health promotion programs—the maintenance of positive health behavior changes. Finally, healthy culture development can support health promotion efforts, increasing the potential for success. Although changing culture is a long-term process, appropriate support enhances employee readiness for behavior change and creates an environment in which it is both acceptable and encouraged.

The four cornerstones of health promotion program development—needs assessment and evaluation, effective intervention, relapse prevention, and healthy culture development—cannot exist without sound administrative procedures and people who will develop and implement those procedures. Perhaps most critical to the overall operation of a worksite health promotion program is the process of attracting, hiring, and training key personnel. The profound changes taking place in the workplace illustrate the importance of aligning health promotion program goals with the business priorities and understanding the relationship between the two. Whether ensuring program growth, program continuance, or the possibility of launching a new business opportunity, there are key critical success factors in the areas of business management, program management, and human resource management that need consideration regardless of how your program's success will be measured.

Part III

Development Strategies for Mature Programs

Part Objectives

Purpose

¬ To provide practitioners of mature programs with insight to new models and applicable case studies.

¬ To provide practitioners of mature programs with more justification for evolving their programs.

Application

¬ All companies are faced with ongoing business challenges. This section provides practitioners with strategies for identifying the health implications from the business challenges.

¬ Battle-tested programs are those that have been in existence for 10 years or longer. Reviewing the case studies from two of these programs will help provide ideas and strategies for mature program practitioners to use immediately.

Vision

¬ Up-to-date resources will help mature program practitioners revitalize and continue to evolve their existing programs.

Chapter 7

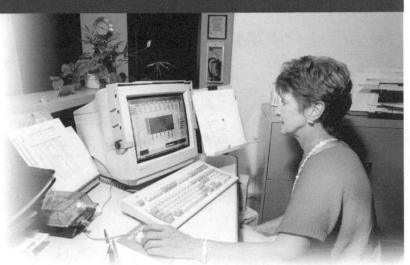

Introducing Development Strategies for Mature Programs

Ask any entrepreneur what period was his or her most exciting time, and he or she will tell you it was growing the business. As the business grows and matures, many entrepreneurs become removed from the things they liked most when they started and are trying to find a way to return to the glory days. Practitioners managing mature programs may have similar thoughts and feelings. The key is to find another aspect of the business that provides the excitement and stimulation of getting started.

Just as businesses go through phases, so do departments and programs. Common themes and principles on which the entity was founded should guide the program or organization through every transition. Two of the key factors that drove every phase, or generation, of worksite health promotion were health outcomes and cost. As initiatives, offerings, and structures have changed, these two factors have been the stimuli.

To put the current state of worksite health promotion in perspective, we must review the various phases that have brought us to this point.

FIRST-GENERATION HEALTH PROMOTION PROGRAMS

In the late 1800s, National Cash Register (NCR) founded what some believe to be the first worksite health promotion program (Chenoweth 1998). NCR wanted to provide its employees with some recreation and leisure activities away from the worksite. Today, we would refer to this arrangement as a recreation program. It may not have been articulated back then, but one can guess that the goals of this program were stress reduction, establishing a sense of camaraderie, and having NCR be seen as a good place to work. Again, one could argue that maintaining health and containing costs were at least partial, if not the only, motivations behind these goals.

SECOND-GENERATION HEALTH PROMOTION PROGRAMS

In the 1970s, several books were released on wellness and aerobics, as were two groundbreaking reports—one in the United States and one in Canada—noting the impact of lifestyle on health and disease. The second-generation of worksite health promotion revolved around fitness. Many companies established fitness facilities at the worksite. The fitness phase recruited more employees and received more attention and backing than the recreation phase. Exercise was considered a way to reduce stress and improve overall health status.

THIRD-GENERATION HEALTH PROMOTION PROGRAMS

In the late 1980s, companies were becoming more sophisticated about health issues. Risk-ful for identification and reduction were the primary driving forces behind this third phase. Many companies today, including mature programs, are still in this phase. Use of the latest intervention strategies and identification techniques further enhances this phase, as does the poor health status of many companies and industries.

FOURTH-GENERATION HEALTH PROMOTION PROGRAMS

The business environment continues to change, and many worksites are becoming less formal. Chief executive officers, especially of high-technology companies, can be seen conducting interviews in casual clothes—something unheard of even 5 years ago. This decrease in formality has also made its way into worksite health promotion. The health and productivity model is seen as the fourth phase of worksite health promotion and is characterized as a new frame of mind that guides program development. Many companies are becoming matrix oriented with emphasis on work teams and cross-functional departments. These characteristics are spilling over into, and in some cases being driven by, worksite health promotion programs.

As you will discover, it is not necessary for a company or program to segment its new fourth-generation model as a stand-alone entity. Core business, specialized company-specific programs, and integration within and across a wide variety of departments are some of the common themes of the fourth-generation model.

THE MATURE PROGRAM

The following chapters are written with the mature program in mind. They are designed to address the current thinking and issues faced by practitioners today, such as the transition to fourth-generation programs mentioned earlier. Another challenge facing mature program practitioners, and practitioners in general, is how to work with managed care organizations. An insightful overview and outlines of specific actions practitioners can take to begin working with managed care organizations are provided.

Benchmarking is a word we hear a lot these days, and Part IV covers this topic, as well as reengineering, in detail. Part IV, however, is also intended for practitioners managing mature programs. Additionally, comprehensive health and productivity management and the work promotion model are described to assist practitioners with organizational improvement. Finally, a summation and the future outlook for mature programs are provided.

SUMMARY

Business reality is demanding that organizations become larger and more comprehensive, yet streamlined. These principles not only apply to core business units within a company but also to all other internal departments and functions. In the past, under the previous three generations of worksite health promotion, integration was viewed as a good thing to do. Now integration is vital to survival. However, accomplishing true integration and understanding all the caveats associated with it is complex. Part III is intended to provide mature program practitioners with ideas and direction on integrating health promotion programs with other important entities.

REFERENCE

Chenoweth, D.H. 1998. *Worksite health promotion*. Champaign, IL: Human Kinetics.

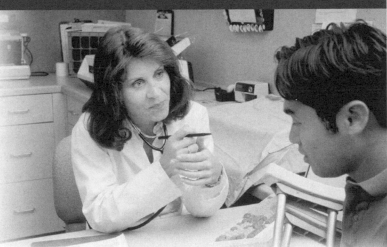

Chapter 8

© Photri, Inc.

Building Partnerships Between Mature Worksite Health Promotion Programs and Managed Care

Mature worksite health promotion programs have a unique opportunity to enhance program outcomes by forming partnerships with the managed care organizations (MCOs) that provide health care coverage for their employees. Such alliances can be especially beneficial to those employers who have large segments of their workforce enrolled in one MCO. However, to create such collaborative approaches to worksite health promotion, a common set of interests needs to be explored, outlined, and agreed on. Ideally, such exploration would be done in a collaborative manner to forge a true partnership. The company and the MCO would be involved in the process to the extent that each has equal power in determining the plan or program, enabling it to negotiate and engage in trade-offs.

INITIAL STEPS TOWARD PARTNERSHIPS

Sometimes companies do not realize the potential of MCO partnerships to enhance their worksite health promotion efforts because of a lack of awareness of the MCO capabilities.

Questions to Ask the MCOs

1. What programs can be made available through the MCO?

    ¬ Primary prevention related

    ¬ Secondary prevention related

    ¬ Tertiary prevention related

    ¬ Catastrophic case management and end-of-life care

    ¬ Managed workers' compensation programs and disability management

    ¬ Centers of excellence for disease-specific care (e.g., cancer treatment, transplants)

2. What is the range of programs (between health promotion and catastrophic case management) that the MCO may be willing to work together on?

    ¬ Screenings

    ¬ Health fairs

    ¬ Risk assessments

    ¬ Disease management

    ¬ Demand management

    ¬ Behavior change programs

    ¬ Rehabilitation services

3. What is the potential for resource leveraging?

    ¬ Time

    ¬ Money

    ¬ Staff

    ¬ Expertise

4. What are the opportunities for additional reach into other community organizations?

   ¬ Additional partnerships brokered by MCO

   ¬ Stakeholders benefited by access to other organizations

5. What data management capabilities are present?

   ¬ Aggregate MCO reports for company executives

   ¬ Employee and dependent data provided to primary care physicians

   ¬ Statistical expertise for creation of analyses and reports

6. What data can be made available for specific populations of interest?

   ¬ Paid claims or claims incurred

   ¬ Code specific (ICD-9, CPT, DRG) health care encounter information

   ¬ Preventable or modifiable portion of total claims dollars

   ¬ Health-risk assessment information

7. How can the data be considered across subpopulations?

   ¬ Employees only (and what proportion)

   ¬ Dependents

   ¬ Early retirees

   ¬ Business unit specific (or bargaining units specific)

8. What kinds of health (risk) assessment tools are already available?

   ¬ Health-risk appraisals (HRAs)

   ¬ Health status assessment (HSAs)

   ¬ Environmental audits and assessments

   ¬ Interest surveys

Although not all of these capabilities may be readily available, they serve as an outline of the possibilities for cooperation. The organizations may decide to combine their efforts toward bringing in additional vendors or other partners so that program components may be linked, leveraged, purchased, or outsourced. Table 8.01 outlines several steps that may be considered as worksite health promotion professionals initiate collaborative relationships with MCOs. What the steps are intended to accomplish, along with additional comments and considerations, is discussed.

It is quite evident from table 8.01 that assessment, identification, and quantification of program impact are important aspects in creating a partnership. Therefore, measurement may be an organizing principle that would allow the stakeholders (employer and MCO) to recognize how and where the program meets mutual and individual goals and objectives.

Measurement of program impact, as a process, allows companies, organizations, and institutions to improve and enhance their capacity and productivity, and to let others know how well they do their business. Measurement cuts across departments, divisions, and business units and even extends beyond the organization into other institutions of the community. It can also outline where similar interests exist and indicate areas of no shared interest. On the other hand, measurement may be inherently limited by the degree to which the collection of variables represents the program scope; that is, if too few aspects of the program are measured, the results may only provide a fragmented and skewed view of what is truly intended to be reported. Hence, the inherent limitations of individual measurements may be offset by a variety of approaches to collecting measurements that may produce sets of data that can create a compelling business case for worksite health promotion programs.

> Employer-based and managed care–based health promotion programs will benefit by fostering creative partnerships that are built around the measurement needs of both organizations and reflect employee and organizational health interest at the same time.

THE NEED FOR DATA

In today's marketplace, organizations are challenged to provide quantifiable means by which they can improve their quality, satisfaction, and productivity. Worksites are aware of the need to ensure a consistent and optimally functioning workforce. Managed care is increasingly held accountable by purchasers of group health benefits, as well as the public, for health care outcomes, especially in the area of quality. Concepts such as total quality management (TQM) and continuous quality improvement (CQI) have been introduced in both worksite and

Table 8.01

Steps to Consider for Creation of a Collaborative Partnership Between Worksite Health Promotion Programs and Managed Care Organizations (MCOs)

STEP	INTENTION	COMMENT
Review of current contract	Understand the limitations of the contract Understand the covered benefits, especially those that impact on the worksite health promotion program components	Prepare thoroughly and be ready to offer suggestions where obvious, or not-so-obvious, opportunities exist
Identify MCO staff and company staff	Work directly with the appropriate MCO staff who have responsibility for the management of the account	The MCO account manager can facilitate an MCO-based project team that includes all expertise needed for the project
Define the target audience	Clear definition of the scope and intended reach of the program	The effort allows for up-front agreement of the scope and provides a denominator for the measurement of the program
Set goals and objectives for the program	Align strategies and measures with the primary purpose of the program Be critical in making sure the program will be cost-consciously implemented	"If you don't know where you're going, any road will get you there." —Pogo, cartoon character
Outline and agree on assessment, monitoring, and measurement approach	Allow for the establishment of a baseline measure Provide opportunity for mutually agreed-upon proportion of the resources applied toward measurement effort Define what will be measured—must be in alignment with the goals and objectives	Should be considered in the context of process, impact, and outcome evaluation Should appropriately consider the culture, environment, and external factors that have an impact on the characteristics (outcome variables) of interest
Agree on ownership and sharing of the results	Understand what will happen to data acquired as part of the program Question and decide who "owns" the data	Considerations should include data confidentiality, anonymity, and privacy In most cases, employers do not want individual level

(continued)

91

Table 8.01

(continued)

STEP	INTENTION	COMMENT
	Question and decide who receives results in aggregate or individual format	data, but aggregate level data that provides understanding of program impact and potential Both parties should receive recognition if results are shared broadly (e.g., in publications)
Agree on approach to cost-sharing, risk-sharing, and benefit-sharing	Specific outline and agreement on resources provided by each of the stakeholders in accordance with the risks and the potential benefits encountered when the program is successful	This step is important because these issues may be difficult to resolve toward the end of the program or in case a program does not follow its intended direction, especially if "scope creep" occurs
Agree on program mix	After an assessment of available evidence for specific program effectiveness, decide what program mix will be most appropriate	Considerations may include cost-effectiveness, method of delivery available and possible, worksite culture, and employee interest
Outline postprogram follow-through on lessons learned, potential for expansion, dissemination of the results, and celebration of the success achieved	Up front, intentionally propose to use this first collaborative program as an example on which a long-term relationship may be built	Without reflection, it is unlikely that a thoughtful postprogram description of lessons learned and appropriate next steps, based on the observed results, will occur successfully

MCO settings to systematically improve performance. Both approaches to quality improvement are data-driven. Although the specific variables of interest may vary between these settings, many of the factors assessed, while described by a different terminology, are actually similar in nature. For example, the employee and dependent in the worksite setting represent a similar demographic variable as the member or patient in the health plan setting.

Similarly, work performance at the worksite may be considered to have comparable characteristics to functional health status as described in a health plan. Reducing time off from work because of illness or injury may

be considered a similar objective to shortening the time to facilitate an employee's return to work from a care delivery system. These measures may serve as examples of the similarity and overlapping interest that both the worksite and the MCO could consider as they work together toward health improvement in a defined population.

In other words, both settings are interested in performance measurement and, hence, are driven by data. The leverage of performance measures represents an enormous opportunity to create synergy between employer-based health promotion programs and managed care–based health management strategies. Therefore, the selection of measures becomes paramount.

Dennis O'Leary, president of the Joint Commission on Accreditation of Healthcare Organizations, reminds us to be cautious: "The problem with measurement is that it can be a loaded gun—dangerous if misused and at least threatening if pointed in the wrong direction." (O'Leary 1995).

Measurement can, however, be responsibly used to paint a true picture of what is to be depicted. The difference between use and misuse may be reflected in the degree to which a set of measures, derived from appropriately implemented data collection techniques, describe the actual state and process that was intended to be measured. To appreciate the notion of measurement, we must understand what measurement can do and what its limitations are.

THE MEANING OF MEASURE

If we consider mature worksite health promotion programs to be comprehensive, we may assume that ongoing measurement and evaluation is an integral component of the program. Furthermore, if we assume that mature programs are able to continually "prove their worth" from a business perspective, the scope of measurement is likely to be broad. The broad scope allows a comprehensive view of the program's impact. This implies that, when considered in total, the individual measures selected as part of the comprehensive measurement and evaluation plan describe the wholeness of the program, but singly, the individual measures represent only fragments of the program. This concept is important. If those fragments do not come together and provide cohesive insight into the essence of the program, then a clear understanding of the program's ultimate goals and its reason for existence will not be achieved. The program itself may well be in jeopardy.

The degree to which a measure represents the total may be expressed through the notion of "ratio." Ratio represents an insight into the proportional relevance of things. "Reason" is derived from the Latin word "ratio." Hence,

consider that if we find a theoretical reason for a worksite health promotion program to exist, we in fact imply that various aspects of the program we describe (its ratio) are all related to what the entire program (the whole) is all about. From this perspective, a thorough understanding of the program fragments we intend to measure will allow us to better understand their relevance to the overall program and the program's relevance to the health of the company. In this context, the notions of measure and ratio provide a subtlety that allows for the description of a program's inherent "healthiness" through the integration and connection of a variety of well-chosen program measurement "fragments." Clarity related to the total impact of the program on the company's health may be brought about by the display of measures in terms of external units as well as through inward reflection of the measures and their meaning within the organization.

THE ROLE OF MEASUREMENT IN STATING THE BUSINESS CASE

Measurement plays a key role in the performance improvement processes of companies and of MCOs. Both entities have extensively invested in the introduction, training, adoption, and continued implementation of CQI and TQM initiatives that are intended to create a constancy of purposeful action toward product and service improvement. The aims of CQI and TQM are directly related to the achievement and maintenance of a competitive advantage in the marketplace as well as the institution of a management style that is collaborative and supportive. Institutional performance may be measured, however, by use of techniques that vary from rigorous research methodology to case study and process descriptions.

Unfortunately, the results obtained after these various approaches to measurement and their interpretations differ inherently. Measurement for improvement will focus on the identification of problems, opportunities for process improvement, and documentation of change in process efficiencies after improvement activities. On the other hand, measurement for research may focus on the pursuit of new knowledge without regard to direct application. It may include complex data collection methodology and thereby exert unacceptable levels of control. It may be extremely expensive and too slow for business objectives to be met. Additionally, in a managed care environment, measurement for accountability tends to be implemented to meet the interests of external parties and is focused on outcomes or results that do not lend insight into the process of improvement itself and may therefore be of limited value for internal purposes.

Although the variety of measurement types and the inherent limitations of each warrant cautious interpretations of results obtained, measurement provides a framework from which a business case may be built that allows for informed decision making at the company executive level regarding health promotion programs. Basically, measurement could be organized in relevance to its role in a research, evaluation, or influence agenda. In this organizing framework, the research agenda represents the most scientifically rigorous measurement approach; the evaluation agenda relates to less rigorous; operationally useful (CQI and TQM) interests, and the influence agenda includes the case examples, the anecdotal evidence, and the personal observation and relevance notion. All three components should be included to make a compelling business case

that leads to a decision-making process favoring the health promotion program.

The business case will also draw on several critical areas or sources of interest. These areas include cost-related aspects (e.g., cost identification, cost effectiveness, and cost-benefit analyses), health-related aspects (e.g., improved health, enhanced functional capacity, and injury reduction), performance-related aspects (e.g., reduced absenteeism, increased alertness, and increased quality), and satisfaction-related aspects (e.g., enhanced morale and positive image). These areas also reflect outcome variables from a measurement perspective. The selection of individual measures should include process, impact, and outcome variables to create a complete measurement profile. Hence, a grid can be constructed that presents the three measurement-related agendas and the four major sources of interest. At any given time, only several cells of the grid may be filled with pertinent data, whereas at other times, all cells may be filled. Taken together, all available single measurement fragments provide the capacity to build a business case that may lead to a decision-making process favoring health promotion. This framework is depicted in figure 8.01.

The framework outlines a grid where a check mark represents the presence of an outcome variable or set of variables related to a specific measurement agenda category. Be-

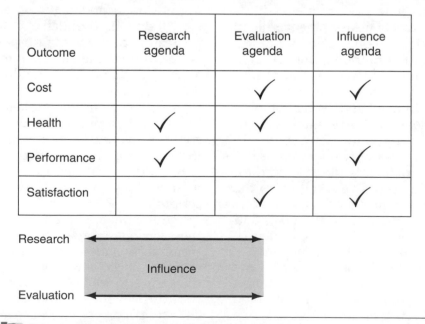

Outcome	Research agenda	Evaluation agenda	Influence agenda
Cost		✓	✓
Health	✓	✓	
Performance	✓		✓
Satisfaction		✓	✓

Figure 8.01 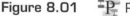 Research, evaluation, and influence agendas.

cause all cells of the grid are in some way meaningfully related to the worksite health promotion program, any cell that contains pertinent data (i.e., any cell that contains a check) may be used to create a business case that better represents the "wholeness" of the program, as opposed to the "fragments" each separate cell represents if considered by itself.

Whereas the research and evaluation agendas are objective in nature, the influence agenda is very subjective. It represents the area where experience and "gut feeling" come into play. It draws on variables that are immeasurable, includes understanding brought about by reflection, and picks up on the right timing. The research and evaluation agendas can be visualized as two parallel lines, and the influence agenda is the space between the lines. As one "reads between the lines," the space allows the meaning to become clear. In such a picture, the space may well be the most important part in bringing comprehension and clarity to a business case. Given such a scenario, a desired outcome may be achieved after the organization's decision-making process.

PARTNERING FOR SUCCESS

Both the worksite and managed care setting have the capacity to clearly define the populations they employ or serve. Health and health improvement are common goals for both parties, and, in the case of mature worksite health promotion programs, the specific populations to be reached at the worksite can be identified and compared with the MCO member population. Once clear goals and objectives have been established, a collaborative approach to improving the health of this defined population makes good business sense for both parties. Setting the goals and objectives, however, may prove difficult if no data are available to outline a case. Data that are available may not be useful unless they have been derived by use of sound measurement and evaluation principles. Hence, measurement may be viewed as a primary opportunity for collaboration between worksite health promotion programs and MCOs.

Much has been written about measurement and evaluation. Many sources are available that outline how to develop an overall evaluation and measurement plan, how to decide what to measure, how to identify the customers of the results, how to select a most appropriate study design, how to write the final report, and so on. Any program can produce reports that make a compelling argument for continuation of a specific aspect of the program. Unfortunately, what impact that particular aspect in the life of a company has on its overall organizational health may not always be clear.

> When worksite health programs are not seen as a major component of the overall health of the company, any measurement or evaluation project by itself will represent no more than a fragment of the larger picture. Therefore, worksite health promotion professionals should periodically take a step back from their daily routines, review the profile of their program, and consider its completeness.

Star Tribune–HealthPartners Worksite Breast Health Management Program Case Study

The following case study is presented as an example of collaboration between an MCO and an employer group with a mature, comprehensive worksite health promotion program. Star Tribune is a newspaper media company with approximately 2,500 employees. HealthPartners is an MCO providing health care coverage for approximately 50% of the employees of Star Tribune and their dependents. The HealthPartners Center for Health Promotion provides worksite health promotion services that are designed to enhance existing company-based programs and integrate health promotion at the worksite with the medical care delivery system. Both organizations are based in Minneapolis, Minnesota.

Background

Star Tribune, after an assessment of their employees' use of preventive health services, was interested in increasing the mammography rate in their group. HealthPartners had previously publicly announced goals that included the intent to increase mammography rates for its membership up to 85%. The initial request was to bring on-site mammography to the worksite. However, mammography is a covered benefit, mobile mammography units are expensive, and nonclinic coordinated screenings do not facilitate performance and accountability measurements for care systems, because these screenings are not documented in the administrative data systems of the MCO or the clinics. Considering these issues, an alternative strategy was sought that would follow sound, evidence-based, best-practice medical care guidelines, would be a systematic means of implementation, would be cost-conscious, and would reach all of its intended audience with minimal disruption of daily operations. Both companies collaboratively designed a more integrated and comprehensive approach.

Setting

The program was implemented in the worksite setting and the clinic setting, and it involved centralized health plan resources to identify individual members and coordinate the overall logistics and information linkages via the Center for Health Promotion staff. The Star Tribune worksite health promotion coordinator worked directly with the Center for Health Promotion worksite health promotion specialist assigned to the program. The Star Tribune provides two health plan options for health care benefits coverage for its employees and their dependents.

Goals and Objectives

The program goal was to design, implement, and measure the impact of a comprehensive breast health management program that in general would reach all female employees and their dependents and in particular focus on the Health-Partners membership for the purpose of increasing compliance with mammography screening guidelines. Specific objectives of the program included

¬ increasing general awareness of breast health issues and knowledge of mammography screening in a defined employee population;

¬ increasing the proportion of female HealthPartners members over age 50

who are in compliance with mammography screening guidelines up to 85% in the defined employee population at this worksite; and

¬ increasing the employer's understanding and awareness of the mammography rate within its own organization.

Implementation

The program had both on-site and off-site components. All on-site components were provided to all Star Tribune employees, regardless of health plan affiliation, and included breast health displays where, at preset times, staff were available for consultation and education. In addition, an "after 40" women's health seminar was held twice during the 6-month program period and was attended by 38 women.

In addition, a letter was mailed to all female HealthPartners members age 40 and older by the MCO. The letter addressed the importance of breast cancer screening, early detection strategies, risk factors, and available resources to reduce identified risks. It also encouraged women age 50 and older to have a mammogram once every 2 years as per medical best-practice guidelines and established Health Plan Employer Data and Information Set measures as released by the National Commission on Quality Assurance. Furthermore, using an innovative, confidential "mammography at-risk registry," the names and phone numbers of all female HealthPartners members age 50 and older who had not received a mammogram within the past 2 years were provided to their health care providers. The health care providers contacted the members by phone and invited them to receive a mammogram (a fully covered benefit).

Results

Of all female employees at the Star Tribune ($N = 888$), 426 were age 40 and older. These 426 women all received the initial letter designed to increase awareness and outline available resources. There were 174 women age 50 and older of which 75% were in compliance with the biennial mammography screening guidelines as indicated by the at-risk lists. Because many women may receive mammograms in settings other than their clinic, the medical records of the 43 women identified on the at-risk list were checked before they were called. Fourteen women had received a mammogram within the past year, and one had undergone a mastectomy. The remaining 28 women received care in 22 different clinics, thus resulting in a request for any given clinic to make no more than four calls. Because of busy clinic schedules, 16 of the 28 calls were completed, and those calls resulted in five mammography appointments. Of the five mammography screenings performed, four were normal and one resulted in detection of early-stage breast cancer.

Hence, the documented biennial mammography screening rate increased by 12% from 75% at the beginning of the project to 87% at the end, thereby exceeding the stated HealthPartners goal of 85%. Furthermore, the early-stage breast cancer detection allowed for early treatment and excellent prognosis. According to published cost estimates for breast cancer treatment, the average 4-year cumulative cost of therapy for early-stage (in-situ, stage I and II) breast cancer is approximately $23,000, whereas the approximate cost of therapy for advanced-stage (stage III and IV) breast cancer is $56,000. Thus, the early detection of one single case of breast cancer represents estimated savings of approximately $33,000 over a 4-year period (average annual savings of $8,250) in direct health care costs. These savings far exceed the cost of implementing the entire program, which was estimated at $2,900. The program was considered to have been cost-consciously implemented and was received with high levels of satisfaction by the employees.

SUMMARY

An external partner, such as an MCO, will likely enhance overall impact of a health promotion program. In such a partnership, both parties play an important role. No one entity can be expected to fix the problems that may exist. Short-term solutions may be used from time to time. However, mature worksite programs must look for long-term, sustainable quality performance while building a culture that cares for its people. After a time of reflection on the company's business interests, the institution's social responsibilities, and the organization's number one asset—its employees—health promotion program partnerships between the worksites and MCOs will make good business sense.

REFERENCE

O'Leary, D.S. 1995. Measurement and accountability: Taking careful aim. *Joint Commission Journal of Quality Improvement* 21:354-357.

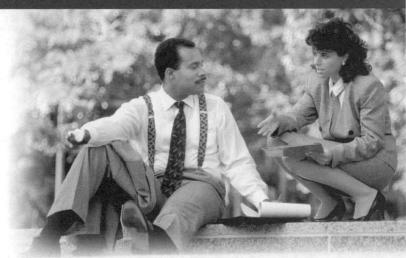

Chapter 9

© N. Bertsch MCMXC

Dow Chemical's Evaluation-Driven Approach

Health promotion at Dow Chemical has been part of the company's Occupational Health Services for almost 7 decades. In 1985, a formal, distinct health promotion program was started at the corporate level. In 1988, this effort evolved to include the creation of a corporate resource center for health promotion, intended to serve the global operations of Dow. Today, health promotion at Dow is administered through the Health Services Expertise Center within the Environment, Health, and Safety Organization. It is part of a number of shared services that are leveraged across the many business units of the company. Health promotion services are intended for Dow families, which include both full-time and part-time employees and their dependents as well as retiree families.

The cornerstone for the success of health promotion at Dow has been the development and application of the Health Promotion Management Standard. A management standard at Dow is used to set the performance requirements and standards by which all Dow sites operate. Management standards exist in a number of other disciplines at Dow, such as Safety and Industrial Hygiene. Although health promotion at Dow has always been data driven, use of the management standard has reemphasized the need for sound evaluation data to drive program development and to show value.

The Dow Health Promotion Vision states that "Health promotion will provide Dow businesses with a competitive advantage through health." This vision implies improved employee health resulting in both enhanced productivity and profitability at the business level as well as increased shareholder value at the corporate level. It also positions Health promotion as an investment strategy rather than purely as an employee benefit. The inherent expectation is that investment strategies are based on sound evaluation methodology.

The three primary objectives (business deliverables) Dow health promotion has established to achieve this vision are

1. improved health status;
2. positive impact on health-related costs; and
3. perception of health promotion as a valued service.

The Health Promotion Management Standard outlines a strategy to ensure these objectives are met. This strategy includes

1. ongoing assessment of the preventive health needs of Dow personnel;

2. maintenance and application of state-of-the-art knowledge of preventive health best practices; and

3. continued program evaluation.

Also inherent to this strategy is ongoing consideration for cost versus impact, materials and interventions based on best practice, and effective utilization of Dow internal and external resources.

Although the planning and evaluation of programs are coordinated through the Health Promotion Resource Center, health promotion at Dow is not an isolated effort. From the beginning, the health promotion staff at Dow has sought and formed relationships with other internal and external partners such as EAP, occupational medicine, industrial hygiene, health care benefits, and safety. This type of integrated approach in planning, implementation, and evaluation has driven many of the preventive health initiatives at Dow. The following initiatives serve as examples of this approach.

Two of the primary health promotion initiatives today at Dow are a result of an extensive review of medical claims, disability claims, and health status data collected in 1996. This review of data led to the development of Dow's Health Targets, which help the company focus its health promotion efforts across North America so that it derives the greatest value and ensures the most appropriate use of its resources. Within Dow, these initiatives are known as "Positive Action" and "The Musculoskeletal Ergonomic Strategy." The following information describes the process of establishing the Health Targets and provides an overview of both of these initiatives.

HEALTH TARGETS

A cross-functional team guided the development of the Health Targets and the strategy to achieve them. The team consisted of representatives from occupational medicine and health promotion. The process involved establishing and assessing quality health target attributes, which helped define the Health Targets and establish outcome goals, influencing factors, process measures and goals, and an implementation strategy.

The resulting Health Targets (see table 9.01) address both supply (prevention) and demand (utilization), and they represent what was felt to be the greatest opportunity to reduce health care costs. The data sources used for establishing these targets included Dow family medical claims, industry-based disability claims from the CDC database, and Dow Employee Health Surveillance data. A decision matrix was used to prioritize preventive health rankings on the basis of their medical claims net cost to Dow, prevalence and cost of unique diagnoses, and severity and frequency of disability incidences.

Use of this decision matrix approach revealed a marked difference between the two top ranked categories, cardiovascular disease and musculoskeletal injury or illness, and the rest. For this reason, these two categories were chosen as the primary preventive Health Targets. On the demand side, an internal "lifestyle claims analysis," combined with the literature, suggested that health care utilization and improved self-management of chronic illness should be the primary objectives and would provide the greatest opportunity to impact health care costs. Interestingly, an analysis of health care claims found similar results

Table 9.01

Health Targets

TARGET	RESULT
Preventive health	Reduce the risk for and incidence of cardiovascular disease
	Reduce risk for and incidence of musculoskeletal injury and illness, on and off the job
Medical consumerism	Improve efficiency of health care utilization
	Improve self-management of chronic illness

in identifying cardiovascular disease, musculoskeletal injuries or illnesses, and medical self-care as three of the top five categories affecting Dow's health care costs.

Once the target areas were established, Outcome Goals (see table 9.02) were determined. These goals refer to changes in medical claims of Dow families and are measured using the health care claims database. Given the lack of historical or long-term data at Dow, the health promotion staff searched the literature for information on the positive effects of risk reduction and made estimates of risk reductions over the next 10-year period. These goals

were realistic, yet challenging, based on a variety of internal factors.

To determine which program development efforts they should focus on to achieve their Outcome Goals, the health promotion staff reviewed the literature to identify factors that were most likely to influence the risk or severity of the target areas. Once again, a decision matrix approach was used to rank the factors in terms of such areas as impact, measurability, data accessibility, prevalence, and value to employees. The result of this analysis is the Influencing Factors (see table 9.03) that help focus and prioritize the health promotion

Table 9.02

Outcome Goals for 2005

TARGET	RESULT
Preventive health	Reduce prevalence of cardiovascular disease medical claims by 5% Reduce prevalence of musculoskeletal injury and illness medical claims by 10%
Medical consumerism	Reduce prevalence of self-care medical claims by 5% Reduce prevalence of chronic illness medical claims by 10%

Table 9.03

Evaluation-Based Program Planning

INFLUENCING FACTORS	PROCESS GOALS FOR 2005	PROCESS MEASURES
PREVENTIVE HEALTH		

Nutritional profile
  Balanced diet
  Fiber intake
  Total blood cholesterol
	Decrease prevalence of borderline-high and high blood cholesterol by 5%; limit increase of overweight population to 30%	Body mass index
		Total blood cholesterol

PHYSICAL ACTIVITY		
Cardiovascular endurance Flexibility Muscular strength and endurance	Increase the population reporting their physical activity at the recommended level by 80%; implement training in 80% of the population	Physical activity level Targeted training Participation

(continued)

101

Table 9.03

(continued)

INFLUENCING FACTORS	PROCESS GOALS FOR 2005	PROCESS MEASURES
PRACTICES AND PROCEDURES		
Inattention or lack of focus Proper practices	Implement awareness and training in 80% of the population	Awareness and targeted training Participation
TOBACCO		
	Reduce the number of persons using tobacco (all forms) by 20%	Reported use of tobacco (all forms)
MEDICAL CONSUMERISM		
Awareness	Provide medical consumerism program access to 100% of Dow families	Medical consumerism program delivery
CONFIDENCE		
	Achieve reported confidence in self-care skills by 85% by Dow families	Reported confidence in self-care skills.
SKILLS		
Chronic illness management Self-care resources	Achieve 25% of individuals with chronic illness participating in intervention	Chronic illness intervention participation Utilization of self-care resources

efforts at Dow. They then set Process Goals based on past experience, as well as what they found in the literature, and Process Measures to evaluate their progress toward these goals.

POSITIVE ACTION

The complete title of this program is *Positive Action: The Wise Health Care Consumer*. This program arose from a comprehensive pilot study conducted at Dow's Michigan operations location in 1994 and 1995. A significant aspect of this study was the program evaluation piece, which was set up to evaluate awareness, knowledge, and confidence in skills as well as the impact on utilization of medical care services. Utilization of program resources was measured through the use of the decision support line and surveys asking the participants which program resources they used. Perception of the program was evaluated through a survey at the 6-month point to determine overall perception of the program, knowledge before and after the program, and confidence in self-care skills. Utilization of medical care services was done through an analysis of claims submissions before and after the program to determine if there was any impact on submission of overall claims, lifestyle-related claims, doctor visits, emergency room visits, hospitalizations, and laboratory and x-ray services.

The overall evaluation of the results of the pilot study showed some positive trends in reduction of total and specific types of claims among participants. Additionally, survey results showed some very positive findings, including 90% of participants who said that Positive Action improved their knowledge as a health care consumer and their communications with their doctor. Also, 89% reported improved self-confidence in home-care skills. Additionally, the program was evaluated on the basis of the return on investment (ROI). Through a reduction of utilization of services, an ROI of 1:1 was seen in the first 9 months after the pilot study. The fact that this reduction was less than what was reported in the literature was offset by the fact that the costs included the installation of a decision support line. Additional evaluation on the indirect cost savings suggested that savings were realized through reduced absenteeism and avoidance of costly medical procedures.

The combination of these results and the data analysis done to establish the Health Targets has driven the design of the key components of this program. The key components of Positive Action are

¬ comprehensive communication strategy;
¬ ongoing evaluation;
¬ action booklets;
¬ self-care triage reference;
¬ family health journal;
¬ decision support line;
¬ Dow Health Information Resource Center; and
¬ chronic illness education.

These components were also driven by an evaluation of both industry best practices and Dow's own claims experience. For instance, one aspect of the chronic illness support is the availability of self-help resources for employees and families that address Dow's top health concerns as identified through internal claims analysis.

Another key to Dow's success has been the fact that the decision support line is funded by the benefits group, and the overall approach is administered through health services (specifically health promotion). In addition, the on-site medical staff plays a key role in promoting the use of this resource through the ongoing health surveillance program as well as through interactions with employees who come into health services for other reasons.

One of the benefits of this approach is the impact of interdepartmental data on benefit plan decisions. For example, the level of coverage from insurance plans for diabetes self-management education can be influenced through high utilization of the demand management line for diabetes-related questions, through prescription trends data from the pharmaceutical prescription administrator, or through information from the internal health surveillance process. Also, this information may drive communication campaigns to increase awareness of the impact of exercise and nutrition on diabetes. Having these data may also help drive targeted interventions to those who need it.

MUSCULOSKELETAL ERGONOMICS STRATEGY (MES)

As in any large manufacturing industry, musculoskeletal injuries and illnesses continue to contribute to higher health care costs and decreased productivity at Dow. Dow Safety and Industrial Hygiene have been tracking incidences and severity (above and beyond OSHA required information), as well as designing strategies to minimize their incidence and impact, for years. At the same time, health promotion has been offering a variety of awareness and educational programs designed to address this need. The data gathered through these efforts, combined with the results of the analysis, led to Dow's Health Targets, resulting in the current cross-functional initiative for managing musculoskeletal disorders.

To address this issue, a team was chartered that was made up of representatives from industrial hygiene, safety, health promotion, and occupational health services. The vision for this team was to create a standardized process that would identify and prioritize key risk factors associated with musculoskeletal injuries and illnesses within Dow and reduce their incidence through prevention and intervention efforts coordinated across health and safety disciplines. The design elements of this strategy included integration of activities at the

Table 9.04

I=P Components of Musculoskeletal Ergonomic Strategy

ACTION	RESULT
Risk identification	Development and identification of tools for self-identification of ergonomic risk and early symptoms
	Delivery mechanism and implementation process
	Data collection and analysis
	Integration with the Dow Health Surveillance
	Program to identify potential at-risk individuals
Intervention efforts	Health counseling for at-risk individuals
	Consultation with plants and businesses on potential administrative and engineering controls, and job restrictions
	Ergonomic related programs and activities offered through health promotion
	Physical preparedness (fitness for duty) programs administered through the occupational health department

local level as guided through a multidisciplinary team, standardizing activities through identification of best practices, and a comprehensive approach to risk control activities. Built into the approach is ongoing data analysis and program validation. The components of this program are found in table 9.04.

SUMMARY

Both Positive Action and the Musculoskeletal Ergonomic Strategy are examples of programs that are driven by evaluation information. Their success lies in the fact that they are per-

ceived as investments in the health of Dow's human assets as well as the fact that they are integrated approaches that require the support and commitment of different departments. Health promotion plays a key role in each of these efforts. To survive and thrive in the corporate environment, Dow must continue to evaluate the effectiveness of its efforts so that it can allocate its resources to where they will have the greatest impact and allow the company to achieve its vision of "providing Dow businesses with a competitive advantage through health."

Chapter 10

© ICS/Photo Network

Implementing Health and Productivity Management

How is increased workforce productivity achieved? Can improvement in the health and well-being of workers result in improved efficiencies? Can human resource professionals develop a business case for investing more in health and productivity initiatives when the overriding business climate is directed at cost cutting? Can the link be made among individual health, organizational health, and overall business performance?

This chapter describes a new and emerging business strategy called health and productivity management (HPM). HPM has become an important focus area for leading-edge organizations seeking to meet their strategic business objectives while managing their total employment costs. These organizations are acutely aware that total employment cost, a major expense item, is a function of several factors: wages, direct benefit costs, and other labor costs.

Q|R Wages include salary, bonuses, stock, savings plans, and commissions. Direct benefit costs, often referred to as fringe benefits, include health insurance, short-term and long-term disability, workers' compensation, and other benefits. Other labor costs, a component that is often overlooked, include the additional human resource costs facing businesses, such as expenses for programs used to increase productivity and morale (e.g., health promotion, fitness facilities, picnics, and other fun events). These costs are important because

of the potential for substantial organizational losses associated with low morale; interpersonal problems; and other physical, mental, or behavioral health problems that influence the productivity of workers and their coworkers.

In short, forward-thinking organizations realize that direct health and disability costs are just the tip of the iceberg. If all the indirect costs are included, such as replacement worker wages, productivity losses, routine overstaffing or overtime premiums, and the intangible costs of dealing with morale issues or interpersonal problems, the effect on organizational performance becomes very significant. With this broad-based view of compensation in mind, innovative organizations are taking steps to proactively manage individual and organizational health to influence bottom-line results (i.e., organizational productivity and profitability).

DEFINING PRODUCTIVITY

What exactly is productivity? In its simplest form, productivity is the number of units produced per person-hour expended. That definition works if you are manufacturing cars or cereal boxes. However, if you are in the computer software, legal, or even medical business, how do you measure the productivity of your workforce?

Think of productivity and productivity loss in two ways:

(1) Productivity is lost when workers are physically absent from work because they are ill, become injured on the job, are subject to a chronic disability, are overcome by stress, or have work-life balance issues. They may be out on short-term or long-term disability; collecting workers' compensation; absent because their child is ill; or experiencing nonmedical, non recreational absence (a real category). They may be taking a family medical leave of absence.

Putting health and disability costs in context, the following factors are exerting significant pressures on American businesses:

¬ Outsourcing, downsizing, and layoffs

¬ Mergers, acquisitions, and consolidations

¬ Global competition

¬ Deregulation

¬ Pressure for innovation, adaptation, and reengineering

¬ Increased reliance on technology

¬ Information overload

(2) The organization may lose worker productivity even if employees are at their desks or workstations. These workers may be physically at work but not "mentally present," or fully functional. They may be suffering from depression, low back pain, allergy, emotional stress, or any number of other physical or emotional conditions. Consequently, these workers are performing at less than peak performance. When you factor in organizational stressors such as downsizing, lackluster senior management, poorly communicated policies, or an environment without clear purpose, productivity losses become even more pronounced. This situation presents a business challenge—not merely a health challenge. The problem is no longer just absenteeism. It's also a problem of "presenteeism."

In addition, many employees are coping with "new work contracts." These contracts send the following messages to workers:

¬ Manage your own career.

¬ Learn new skills in order to remain "marketable."

¬ Share in the costs.

¬ Take ownership of the organization's success.

¬ Only the fittest survive.

How have employees responded to these pressures? Some thrive. They become entrepreneurs, intrapreneurs, team leaders, innovators, and change agents. Domino's Pizza became a success because the owner brought the store to you knowing that you were too busy to go out and get the pizza yourself. Wal-Mart became the dominant retailer because it provided variety, low cost, and customer service. Fed eral Express created a demand for overnight package delivery, a service that did not exist 30 years ago.

Whereas some employees have thrived, others have suffered under these pressures. Their response has included burnout, lack of commitment, feelings of instability, and a reexamination of career decisions.

Job and personal stresses have manifested themselves as medical, psychological, behavioral, and organizational symptoms reflecting increased health and productivity risks. These risks are

¬ medical, including chest and back pain, heart disease, gastrointestinal disorders, headaches, dizziness, weakness, and repetitive motion injuries;

¬ psychological, including anxiety, aggression, irritability, apathy, boredom, depression, loneliness, fatigue, moodiness, and insomnia;

¬ behavioral, including accidents, drug and alcohol abuse, eating disorders, smoking, tardiness, "exaggerated" disease; and

¬ organizational, including absence, poor work relations, turnover, low morale, job dissatisfaction, and low productivity.

FRAGMENTED ORGANIZATIONAL STRUCTURES

In most organizations, the various types of risk are handled separately and discreetly by different parts of the organization, such as employee benefits, employee assistance programs, risk management, occupational medicine, safety, organizational development, operations, human resources, employee relations, and labor relations. However, risks are often common to several areas of the organization and could be better managed via cooperative or higher-level endeavors rather than by fragmented, department-specific strategies (see figure 10.01).

In a hierarchical structure, each organizational function attempts to handle company-wide issues using a variety of interventions, including

¬ managing disability;

¬ managing health care;

¬ managing demand for health care and disease;

¬ managing stress;

¬ strengthening employee assistance programs;

¬ reengineering;

¬ reorganizing;

¬ providing incentives;

¬ penalizing certain behaviors;

¬ training staff;

¬ cutting costs; and

¬ introducing new initiatives.

Do any of these intervention programs work? The jury is still debating the effectiveness of these intervention programs because there are relatively few published studies evaluating program outcomes. Nonetheless, most, if not all, of these intervention strategies are firmly embedded in most American businesses.

COST MANAGEMENT—A HISTORICAL PERSPECTIVE

If we turn back the clock and focus on effective cost-management strategies implemented during the 1980s, we see that they can be grouped into three main categories. First, health care purchasers (employers) shifted more of their costs to their employees, thus making employees more sensitive to the cost burden associated with medical care. Additionally, employers held employees more accountable for paying a greater proportion of medical expenditures. This cost shift occurred primarily through development of new benefit plan designs that introduced higher deductibles, coinsurance payments, and larger out-of-pocket ceilings. Newer plan designs such as medical savings accounts (MSAs) have further shifted responsibility for medical payments to consumers of health services.

Second, purchasers aggressively negotiated discount and creative fee payment arrangements with providers and health plans that were based on diagnosis-related groups (DRGs), resource-based relative value scales

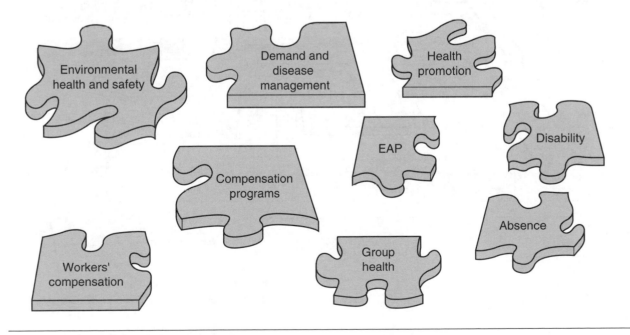

Figure 10.01 Common approach—individual program management.

(RBRVS), and various capitation schemes. Health maintenance organizations (HMOs), preferred provider organizations (PPOs), point of service (POS) plans, exclusive provider organizations (EPOs), and other alternative funding plans were developed, all of which fell under the broad banner of managed care.

Third, purchasers introduced vigorous utilization management programs whose aims were to reduce the number and length of hospitalizations and prevent unnecessary or inappropriate care. These intervention programs worked well individually or in combination to reduce excess health care utilization and cost. Perhaps they worked too well, given the current backlash against managed care.

SOLUTIONS FOR THE CURRENT ERA

What is different today? For one thing, more attention is being directed at quality of care and outcomes of treatment—dimensions of care that may have been neglected in a zeal to contain costs. Most recently, employers are requiring their health plans to identify and codify best-practice guidelines for managing patients with acute and chronic conditions and to monitor adherence to these guidelines as a matter of protocol. Also, there is a growing recognition that health and productivity are interrelated and that more emphasis must be placed on prevention and health promotion.

We find that our daily experience, especially our ability to balance work and family life, is becoming far too complicated (see figure 10.02).

At an organizational level, we live in a fragmented, uncoordinated organizational web where every department has its own turf, its own fiefdom, and its own silo. We attack problems individually, one at a time, and in an uncoordinated fashion. We need a new way to think about organizational problems and develop increased efficiencies for addressing a more complex landscape (see figure 10.03).

AN INTEGRATED MODEL

HPM establishes a new paradigm for working across departments and functions

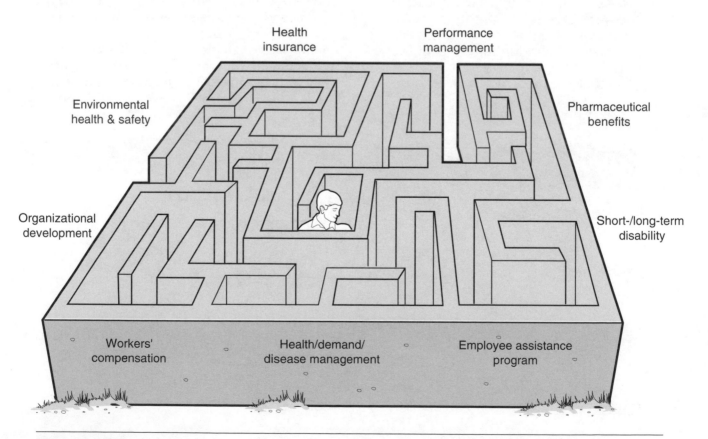

Figure 10.02 The reality—life is getting very complicated.

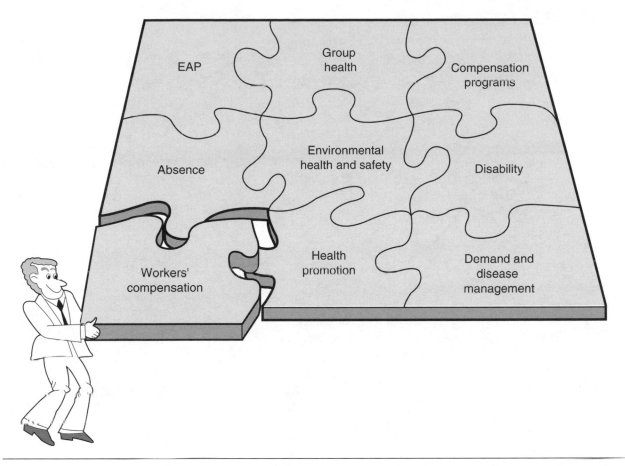

Figure 10.03 Health and productivity management—putting the pieces together.

to put all the pieces together to form a coordinated, synergistic, and unidirectional set of solution packages. The aim of HPM is to move toward an integrated approach that is focused on people, not cases, regardless of where corporate programs reside. A synergistic team aims to coordinate care across common providers, across common conditions, across benefit plans, and across locations.

> Because of resource constraints and increasing complexities associated with program and people management, departments cannot afford to do their job in piecemeal fashion anymore. They need to get "all hands on deck" working together to achieve an optimal balance between people needs and business needs.

HPM—A PRACTICAL APPROACH

How, then, is this balance accomplished? Figure 10.04 presents a schematic diagram of a process for implementing HPM. First, a cross-functional HPM team needs to establish where the organization is at greatest risk—peoplewise, programwise, or expensewise. This determination is made through a diagnostic assessment of organizational and individual health. Then, colleagues should meet to prioritize identified problems and form a strategic action blueprint. Next, the group should design and implement a set of solutions—packages of solutions, not individual programs. The organization should then evaluate whether the packages of solutions achieved their intended results. Finally, managers should act on the recommendations made during the evaluation process to strengthen weak but useful programs, expand beneficial programs, and replace programs that are clearly not effective.

Undergirding this entire process are available, reliable, and actionable data. A critical first step in developing an HPM strategy is to gather the disparate data that are scattered

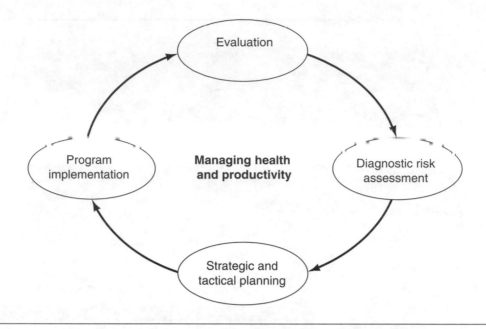

Figure 10.04 Health and productivity management approach.

across the organizational landscape and bring them all together. Connect the dots by connecting the data by person, provider, condition, plan, and location. The idea is to perform a physical and psychosocial examination of your organization to diagnose where the risks to health and productivity exist so that effective action can be taken. Next, it is helpful to compare the organization's experience with norms and benchmarks. This comparison will help determine whether your experience is in the good (white), average (dotted), or below average (shaded) zone by HPM category (see figure 10.05).

Next, examine the dollars spent on employees not only within the program but also holistically, across programs. How are those dollars distributed? Where are the biggest expenses, and where are the biggest opportunities? Compare the organization's metrics with benchmarks. Calculate savings opportunities on the basis of the difference between current metrics and judgments about how closely the organization should be able to match benchmarks. Further diagnostic work should direct you to the "drivers" for high cost and low productivity (see figure 10.06). For example, look for the overlap in the use of company programs. Is a relatively small group of employees or business units accounting for relatively high utilization in multiple programs (e.g., medical benefits, disability programs, employee assistance programs)? Why is their program utilization high?

HPM Case Study

Some case study examples will illustrate the type of detective work done to uncover HPM opportunities.

Case Study 1

Company A examined the number of days employees took off for nonrecreational (vacation, holiday) activities. Most employees took a reasonable number of days off (less that 15 days/year), but 28% of employees accounted for 80% of the total days taken. In fact, more than 300 employees in the company took more than 200 days off per year out of an available 225 days (see figure 10.07). Senior management's immediate response was predictable: "Why are these people still on our payroll?" The answer was that some of these employees were absent for very legitimate reasons, whereas others were suffering from less tangible conditions such as "stress" or "pain."

Figure 10.08 represents the "Pareto group" of employees from this company, the group that comprised 20% of the highest-cost employees in the organization. The Pareto group accounted for about 80% of incidental absences, 40% of medical costs, 65% of short-term disability payments, and 40% of workers' compensation

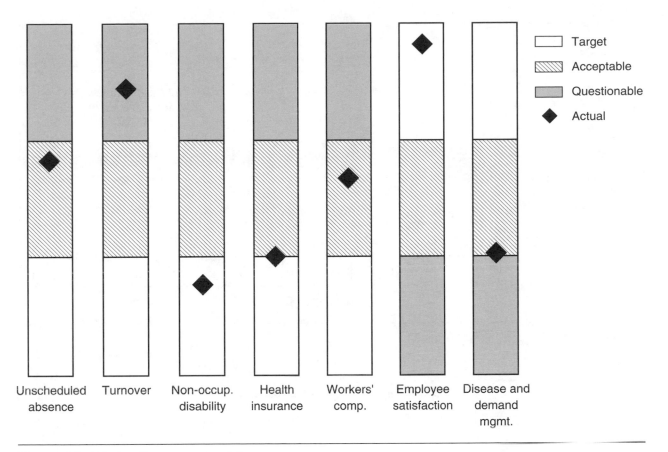

Figure 10.05 Quality program risks.

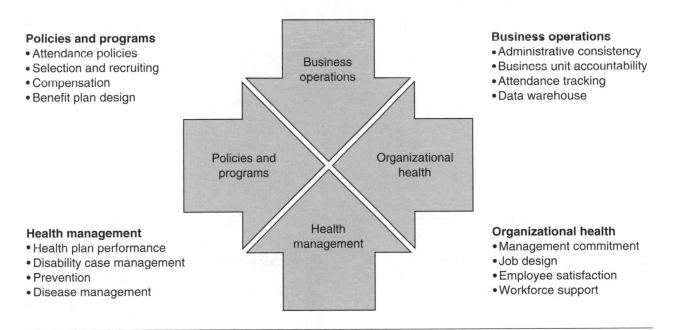

Figure 10.06 Health and productivity management drivers.

111

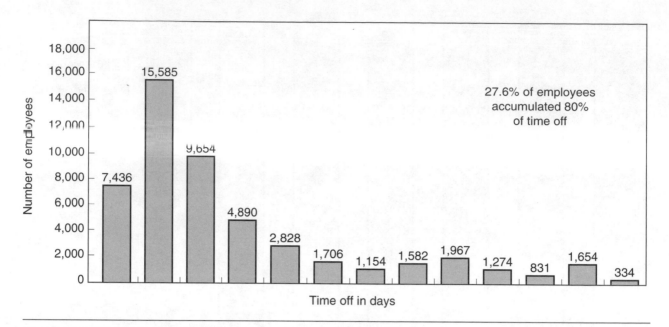

Figure 10.07 Time-off experience.

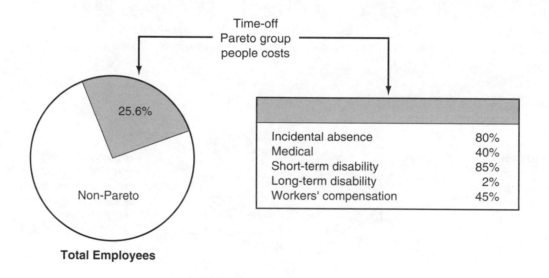

Figure 10.08 Pareto maldistribution and overlap.

costs. Their average group health costs were about $12,000/claimant, workers' compensation costs were $2,000/claimant, and disability program costs were $9,000/claimant. All together, these Pareto group employees cost the company about $23,000 a year, about three times the total health and productivity management costs for the average employees. In response, the company decided to focus on employees and conditions that were most costly while introducing better health and disease management protocols for all employees. The focused effort resulted in cost savings and improved worker productivity.

Case Study 2

Figure 10.09 depicts the results of a study performed with a large multinational con-

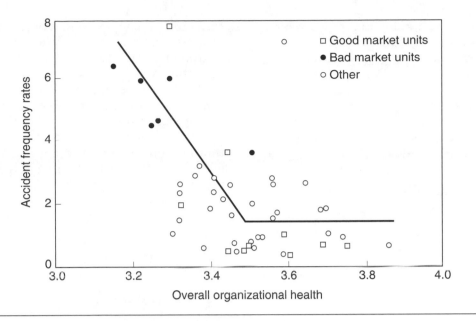

Figure 10.09 The "kink" of organizational health.

glomerate. An analysis uncovered, almost accidentally, a clear relationship between organizational health, as measured in an annual company-wide employee opinion survey, and the number of on-the-job accidents, or accident frequency rate. If organizational health fell below a certain value (i.e., 3.5 on a 1 to 5 scale), accidents increased significantly for any given business unit. The analysis documented the cost of poor organizational health and its impact on accident rates and workers' compensation claims. In this case, the company focused attention on improving the culture and climate at key locations. This intervention subsequently improved the accident frequency rate and cost experience at those locations.

The work world is changing rapidly. Organizations are beginning to focus on improving profitability and increasing productivity. One avenue for improving productivity is keeping workers on the job by preventing diseases and accidents, limiting the time for disability, providing a healthy organizational culture, and keeping employees motivated. The human resources departments' role has evolved from being a cost center to being a catalyst for change. They recognize that individualized, independent, and uncoordinated approaches no longer make sense. What is needed is a comprehensive integrative model of health and productivity management that considers individual, organizational, and societal influences on health and productivity.

Innovative managers can implement HPM within their organization by doing the following:

1. Along with their colleagues in different sections of the organization, commit to a collaborative approach to solving common, organization-wide problems and improving the work culture.

2. Effectively diagnose HPM-related problems that run across departments (e.g., job stress, physical health problems, mental and behavioral problems, and organization malaise). Also, bring forward examples of best practices that should be emulated organization-wide.

3. Determine the root sources of organizational problems (the "drivers") through effective quantitative and qualitative data analysis.

4. Work together with fellow managers to identify potentially useful methods for addressing the problems by using "solution packages" delivered in an integrated rather than a silo fashion.

5. Implement the program packages effectively by using best-practice and state-of-the-art methods.

6. Track, monitor, and evaluate the intervention programs rigorously.

7. Learn from the evaluations to fine-tune and correct program deficiencies.

SUMMARY

Improving the bottom line of an organization involves having a positive impact on issues such as employee health, morale, and something amorphous called culture and values. Because workers are truly an organization's most important assets, there is a strong need to attend to their personal issues and the associated issues of organizational health. Managers and workers should promote a healthy company culture because the payback is significant, both in terms of finances and in terms of intangible factors such as improved morale. Improvement in the health and well being of employees makes a company a better, more productive place to work.

Chapter 11

Improving the Organization Through the Work Promotion Model

The reality of today's business environment requires the flexibility and agility of a gymnast to rapidly respond to the demands (e.g., from customers, competitors, and investors) of a changing marketplace. However, no matter how well systems are designed and implemented to promote continuous quality improvement or how lean and mean an organization may become, there remains a central core of human capital responsible for creating, planning, producing, selling, servicing, and administering the business. Human capital will remain the core asset of every sustainable organization. Therefore, the health promotion manager must offer initiatives that address not only the cost concerns of the organization but also the quality-of-life concerns of the individual employee (Pfeiffer 1998).

WORK PROMOTION AND WORK ECOLOGY

Within this context, targeted worksite health promotion initiatives are not health promotion per se but work promotion activities. Work promotion can be defined as organizational supports and activities that protect, support, and enhance human capital in the fulfillment of meaningful employment and meaningful profits. Work promotion is part of a much broader concept called work ecology—the interactions among the organization, individuals, and work groups within the total business environment. Work ecology strives to create and sustain

Work Promotion Versus Health and Productivity Management

Whereas work promotion is concerned with managing human capital to minimize relevant risks and costs and their impact on work performance and overall productivity, health and productivity management (HPM) provides the tools and processes to measure and quantify the influence of these factors on business outcomes. In human capital management, people and "people factors" (e.g., health status, job competency, presence, output, and motivation) are the focus of work promotion activities.

Therefore, improving business performance requires more than lowering the direct costs of health benefits. There is a performance line in addition to a cost line, and creating value to the organization requires paying attention to both. Health and productivity management helps identify and define these value propositions. In the human capital model, the following statements apply:

1. Managing your corporate benefits should not constitute a set of practices separate and apart from managing your workforce.
2. People are the focus. Healthy, at-work, and optimally functional employees use fewer benefits and are more productive.
3. For employer–health plan partnerships to be successful, the value and management functions pursued jointly must solve both direct and indirect costs of ill health.

balanced performance systems that benefit not only the organization and its employees but also its customers, its stockholders, and the communities they serve without creating harm directly or indirectly to those related to the enterprise. Balanced performance systems attempt to optimize and target resources (e.g., capital, employees, and raw materials) in achieving the primary goals of profitability and employability.

The role of the health promotion manager within this model is multifaceted and cross-functional. The health promotion manager is part of a human capital team (HCT) that is composed of human resource–related functions whose mission is to create and sustain a balanced work environment that supports both the organization's business objectives and the individual's needs.

THE WORK PROMOTION MODEL—MANAGING TWO PERSPECTIVES

Within the work promotion model, meaningful profit and meaningful employment not only coexist but also are interdependent. The employer and employee have a social contract with each other in which each side is mutually responsible for the success of the other. The role of the health promotion manager and the HCT is to align and integrate their respective ser-

The Work Promotion Model

Managing risk and its related costs is the most expedient way for human capital managers to align their services with the business goals of their organizations. Within this context, risk is not limited to health risks and their associated costs. It also includes absenteeism, occupational illness and injury, disability, and other factors that undermine total productivity and the bottom line. For example, presenteeism—diminished work capacity related to such factors as chronic illness and work-life conflicts—has significant impact on productivity and its associated costs. Therefore, health management needs to be positioned as part of a broader, more integrated approach to risk management or, in other words, work promotion (see figure 11.01).

Work promotion is defined as organizational initiatives that protect, support, and enhance human capital in the fulfillment of the following goals:

¬ Enhanced health and productivity of the workforce

¬ Improved employability (value) of the workforce by the acquisition of skill sets that also include appropriate work-care and self-care practices

¬ Sustained profitability and growth to the organization and its shareholders

The bottom line is healthier profits and a healthier, more productive workforce.

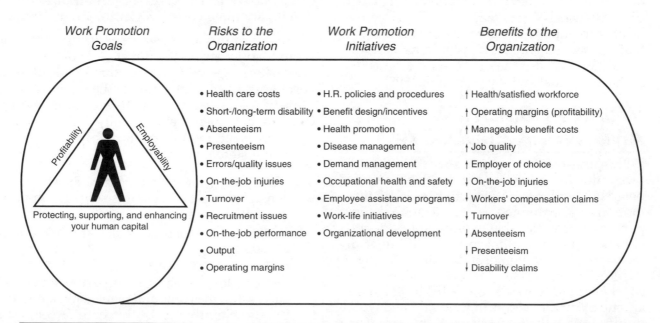

Work Promotion Goals	Risks to the Organization	Work Promotion Initiatives	Benefits to the Organization
Profitability / Employability — Protecting, supporting, and enhancing your human capital	• Health care costs	• H.R. policies and procedures	↑ Health/satisfied workforce
	• Short-/long-term disability	• Benefit design/incentives	↑ Operating margins (profitability)
	• Absenteeism	• Health promotion	↑ Manageable benefit costs
	• Presenteeism	• Disease management	↑ Job quality
	• Errors/quality issues	• Demand management	↑ Employer of choice
	• On-the-job injuries	• Occupational health and safety	↓ On-the-job injuries
	• Turnover	• Employee assistance programs	↓ Workers' compensation claims
	• Recruitment issues	• Work-life initiatives	↓ Turnover
	• On-the-job performance	• Organizational development	↓ Absenteeism
	• Output		↓ Presenteeism
	• Operating margins		↓ Disability claims

Figure 11.01 The work promotion model.

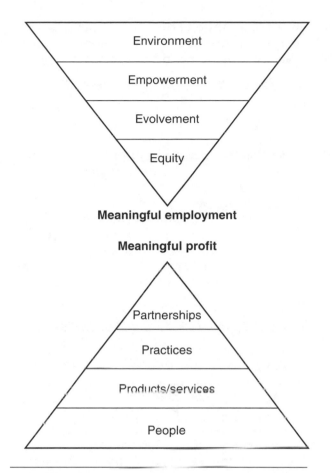

Figure 11.02 Double pyramid.

vice offerings in the program levels that are most appropriate to their capabilities and to the mission and goals of the HCT. As figure 11.02 illustrates, the work promotion model is depicted as two pyramids with four interrelated levels that meet at their apex.

THE ORGANIZATION'S PERSPECTIVE— MEANINGFUL PROFIT

As outlined, the organization's primary goal is to produce and sustain meaningful profit that is aligned with its mission. To attain this goal, four interrelated factors must work in synchrony: people, products and services, practices, and partnerships.

MEANINGFUL PEOPLE

Be it a two-person shop or a multinational corporation employing tens of thousands of workers, having the right people with the right competencies (skills and attitudes) is the foundation of any successful enterprise. For it is people who bring value to the organization, contributing individually and as a group to its short-term and long-term success.

MEANINGFUL PRODUCTS AND SERVICES

From the minds and hands of an organization's people come the innovation and effort to produce products and services that meet specific needs and have a perceived value by the marketplace. However, a key success factor of a sustainable organization is its ability to continuously renew (Gnoshal and Bartlett 1997) itself through innovation and an entrepreneurial spirit.

MEANINGFUL PRACTICES

Organizations can have meaningful people and meaningful products or services, but unless there is a process that maintains excellence (quality) and efficiencies (costs), even the best companies can quickly lose customer loyalty and market share. Successful organizations embrace and follow the concept of best practices, policies, systems, and processes that strive to do such things as reduce the time to create and commercialize products, reduce defects and errors, improve customer support, and reduce product costs to improve overall quality.

MEANINGFUL PARTNERSHIPS

The last level from the employer's perspective is the creation, expansion, and maintenance of meaningful partnerships. These relationships are internal and external to the organization. They include the interactions of

¬ employees;

¬ work teams; and

¬ the organization.

For example, the expanding role of managed care plans in assuming health promotion activities to their respective members (employees) can be viewed as a threat to the health promotion manager. However, the opportunity to identify (benchmark) programs that, as discussed earlier, develop products and services that serve the needs of one's internal customers (partners) is a critical success factor for human capital managers.

Key attributes of meaningful partnerships between human capital functions and their end users include

¬ easy access to products and services;

¬ a level of trust and comfort between involved parties;

¬ guaranteed confidentiality;

¬ demonstrated credibility and professionalism;

¬ genuine caring and empathy; and

¬ appropriate follow-up.

> Maximizing the value of each level of this model not only improves the likelihood of business success by better positioning and improving the value of the organization's human capital but also improves the likelihood of employees developing their own capabilities.

THE EMPLOYEE'S PERSPECTIVE— MEANINGFUL EMPLOYMENT

Q R As reported in *Fortune* magazine (Grant 1998), the Gallup Organization conducted a survey of 55,000 workers on the correlation between job attitudes and company performance (profits). Four key attitudes were found to have the strongest correlation with profits:

¬ Workers feel they are given the opportunity to do what they do best every day.

¬ They believe that their opinions count.

¬ They sense that their fellow workers are committed to quality.

¬ They make a direct connection between their work and the company's mission.

The factors that contribute to meaningful employment and one's employability are meaningful environment, meaningful empowerment, meaningful evolvement, and meaningful equity, as described in the following sections.

Meaningful Environment

R To the average worker, the foundation of meaningful employment is belonging to a meaningful work environment. The place of one's work can be a crucible in which ideas and energy react to create new forms (opportunities) or only a furnace that burns away initiative.

Meaningful Empowerment

Empowerment can be defined as the latitude to exercise decisions within one's work role. Empowerment is not only organizational license to take ownership of one's job but also the capability to take ownership. License is meaningless unless the worker has the proper skills and support in place. Perhaps there is no greater area where empowerment can be manifested than in the area of personal health. Health promotion activities are empowering abilities that demonstrate self-mastery, which are then transferable to other areas of one's work and life.

Meaningful Evolvement

Q Our work, what we do, ideally evolves over the course of our career(s) as we go from apprentice to tradesman to master. Schumacher (1973) calls it perfecting our gifts. In turn, the feeling that employees are recognized for making a difference is perhaps the strongest predictor of job satisfaction. Therefore, providing the opportunity for continuous learning is a major factor not only for protecting one's skills but also for enhancing employability. Within health promotion, the evolvement of the physical self is a self-affirming experience to many employees who have not paid attention to their physical needs, and it further reinforces self-management and personal empowerment.

Meaningful Equity

The last factor within this model is meaningful equity. Equity means a level playing field, an environment of fairness and trust. Additionally, equity is a product of empowerment and involvement. It is a positive return on investment that says: "My work has value." Finally, there is another dimension of equity that is often not discussed within business circles but is perhaps a major factor in the dissonance between one's work and personal life. It is the perceived absence of spiritual equity. Fox (1995), in his book *The Reinvention of Work*, eloquently discusses the rift between work and life in general: "Life and livelihood ought not be separated but to flow from the same source, which is Spirit, . . . both life and livelihood are about living in depth, living with meaning. . . and a sense of contributing to the greater community. A spirituality of work is about bringing life and livelihood back together again." Work promotion initiatives can contribute to all dimensions of equity by initiating supports that protect and enhance the quality of one's work life.

PUTTING THE MODEL TO WORK

The model not only presents a framework for optimizing human capital and the overall value of the organization but also purports to be a philosophy of work. Because this model is multidimensional, it needs to be multifunctional. As discussed earlier, health promotion managers cannot function within a program vacuum. They need to be strategically aligned with related human resource functions through the development of an HCT.

The HCT represents a cross-section of managers involved in the management of human capital issues. The members believe that an organization's total value begins and ends with quality people. The members accept that personal effectiveness and productivity is a product of the total person. The team's purpose is to provide quality services that have an impact on profitability and employability. These services can be placed under three general categories whose functions are to protect, support, or enhance the capabilities of individuals and work teams to make better work-related decisions that minimize risk, improve business outcomes, and create an environment that encourages employability.

WORKSITE HEALTH PROMOTION'S ROLE

The director of the worksite health promotion program should take a focal role in assembling and implementing the HCT. If a worksite health promotion program is just being started, the assembly of the HCT should occur during the time that the needs assessment is being conducted. In the case of a more seasoned program, if a needs assessment has been conducted recently, then the results only need to be reviewed in preparation for putting the HCT together.

In any case, the assembly and implementation of an HCT involves the following four steps:

Step 1—Assess the Organization for the First Time or Use the Results of an Organizational Study That Has Been Completed

¬ Examine the structure of the organization and identify the various business units and departments, decision-making chain of command, and budget centers.

¬ Examine the organization's mission, overarching goals, and corporate philosophy or culture. Review internal documents and interview management and employees to become acquainted with the nature of the organization's business. When talking to managers, determine what their employee-related issues are. Find out what is working and what is not working. Ask them how they think you can help them overcome some of these challenges. Be sure to start with top-level management. These individuals frequently have final say on budgets, and if you are successful in getting their support, other managers will tend to follow.

¬ Identify the key internal and external departments, vendors, people, and programs that provide health-related services for the organization. This group may include internal entities such as medical and health services, benefits department, occupational health and safety, disability management, and training and development. External vendors may include employee assistance programs, managed care organizations, and vendors who provide specific services such as 24-hour nurse lines, prenatal programs, or health-risk appraisal services.

¬ Determine the function and scope of services provided by these groups by reviewing internal documents, attending meetings, and interviewing key players.

Step 2—Determine How Worksite Health Promotion Fits Within the Organization

¬ Review all human capital services and programs provided by internal and external groups.

¬ Create a cross-functional matrix that identifies unique contributions, opportunities, redundancies, and gaps in delivery of health-related services by the various organizations.

¬ Determine potential for worksite health promotion to connect with internal and external groups in provision of delivery of human capital services and programs. For instance, different groups may offer similar services (e.g., health screenings, stress management programs, and back pain management services).

Step 3—Assemble the HCT

¬ Examine the results of the organizational assessment and cross-functional matrix.

¬ Identify representatives from the various internal and external groups who are key to operationalizing the work ecology framework in accordance with organizational goals and strategies.

¬ Determine strategies to raise awareness and educate these representatives about the work ecology philosophy and the need to create an HCT.

¬ Invite identified constituents to serve on the HCT. Conduct an initial meeting to discuss opportunities for collaboration. You may need to start slow as issues may present significant challenges. However, continue to articulate the vision and encourage an integrated approach.

Step 4—Implement the HCT

¬ Work with team members to identify key issues and challenges faced by the organization that affect the profitability and employability goals. Analyze medical and workers' compensation claims and injury and accident rates. This information will provide insight as to specific business risks. For instance, are workers' compensation claims increasing? Is slumping morale affecting work quality and output?

¬ Study best practices of sister organizations relative to these human capital issues and challenges. This benchmarking approach commonly provides ideas and methodologies to improve specific functions and offers criteria to plan and measure progress.

¬ Develop an integrated approach that optimizes cross-functional synergies and pools resources. Determine specific initiatives, goals, and strategies to be undertaken. Demographics, health trends, risk data, and cultural readiness should be used to provide further information and direction.

¬ Appoint team leaders for each initiative on the basis of the team members' expertise and focus.

¬ Clarify the roles and responsibilities of each HCT member relative to each objective.

¬ Encourage cross-functional problem solving and project ownership.

¬ Determine evaluation strategy on the basis of well-defined performance benchmarks that relate to principal goals and strategies.

¬ Monitor progress on a regular basis and modify plans and strategies as needed.

¬ Communicate regularly with and maintain support and involvement of management.

SUMMARY

The establishment of an HCT is a significant task, especially within large organizations where turf issues may be not only personality differences but also cultural differences. HCT development needs to be sanctioned by senior management as a standing committee that operates on an ongoing basis. Its two primary goals, as reiterated throughout this section, are to enhance organizational profitability and employability by optimizing the value of its people.

REFERENCES

Fox, M. 1995. *The reinvention of work*. New York: HarperCollins.

Gnoshal, S., and C. Bartlett. 1997. *The individualized corporation: A fundamentally new approach*. New York: HarperCollins.

Grant, L. 1998. Happy workers, high returns. *Fortune* 137, 81-84.

Pfeiffer, G. 1998. Work promotion vs. health promotion: Aligning your services with the needs of the organization and its people. *Worksite Health* 1, 14-20.

Schumacher, E.F. 1973. *Small is beautiful*. London: Abacus.

Chapter 12

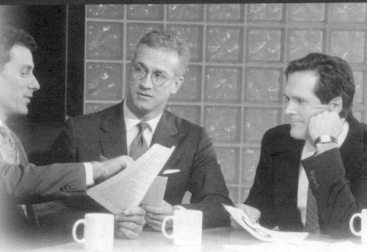

© ICS/Photo Network

Presenting Final Thoughts for Mature Programs

Given the ever-changing nature of corporate America, one thing is certain: Mature worksite health promotion initiatives of the twenty-first century are going to be very different from the ones we knew in the twentieth century. Events such as the globalization of our economy, an increasing reliance on technology, the escalating costs of health care, and profound demographic changes—not to mention the very real pressures to demonstrate tangible and visceral improvements to the company's bottom line—all contribute to the need for new and different approaches to worksite wellness in mature programs. In an attempt to help practitioners and researchers successfully meet the demands and challenges of the future, we have provided several "final thoughts" for consideration.

Specifically, we have identified four issues that merit serious consideration. They include

¬ increasing senior-level support;

¬ clock building versus time telling;

¬ developing key organizational health indicators; and

¬ broadening the understanding of the actual determinants of health.

Certainly, this list is not meant to be comprehensive. However, we are confident that, if those charged with leading mature health promotion programs address each one of these four issues, their programs will be substantially more effective.

Although these final thoughts are most assuredly guided by the research, they are admittedly less about the hard science of worksite health promotion and more about the "art of the possible." They are, in essence, a collection of thoughts and ideas intended to stimulate and inspire those who have been charged with leading mature worksite wellness programs into the future to become the architects of nothing less than world-class wellness initiatives.

INCREASING SENIOR-LEVEL SUPPORT

Effective worksite wellness initiatives—especially in mature programs—require the complete and unwavering support of senior corporate officers. Although much has been written about the importance of enlisting the support of senior executives, it still remains somewhat of an elusive proposition for many wellness professionals. To be sure, only a fortunate few can boast of strong support from the corner office—support that is characterized by more than just a casual interest and "management by abdication."

The first item that should be given serious consideration by those who have been charged with leading mature wellness initiatives is the urgent need for increasing the amount of senior-level support.

What roles should senior-level officials be expected to assume in the delivery of these important initiatives? Five key roles that senior-level executives can and should assume in moving the worksite wellness initiative forward are suggested (Hout and Carter 1995; Chapman 1997; Elliott 1998; Heifetz and Laurie 1997). These roles include

¬ communicating the vision;

¬ providing a positive role model;

¬ allocating adequate resources and initiating supportive policies; and

¬ recognizing and rewarding employee success.

While it is beyond the scope of this discussion to elaborate on these roles, it is sufficient to say that senior-level leadership in mature wellness initiatives cannot be a rare event or a once-in-a-lifetime proposition. As a result, if mature worksite wellness initiatives are to grow and prosper in the future, those professionals responsible for shepherding the wellness initiative will need to obtain more meaningful support from senior-level executives if they hope to be effective.

CLOCK BUILDING VERSUS TIME TELLING

Although enlisting the support of senior-level leaders is important, it certainly is not the only concern for mature programs. A second issue that deserves consideration is the challenge of enlisting others throughout the organization in embracing the concept of worksite wellness.

Indeed, in their insightful book *Built to Last*, organizational researchers James Collins and Jerry Porras (1997) explored the phenomenon of how some companies have been able to survive and excel for the better part of the twentieth century, despite overwhelming circumstances and a brutally competitive business environment. Early in the book, the authors brought to the forefront the organizational concept of clock building versus time telling. According to Collins and Porras (1997), time telling refers to those rare gifted leaders who are both visionary and charismatic—the kind of leaders who almost single-handedly take charge to make good things happen within an organization.

Contrary to the idea of time telling is the notion of clock building. Clock building is the arduous practice of melding the gifts and tal-

ents of individuals throughout each of the company's strategic areas in an effort to build an organization that can prosper far beyond the presence of any single leader. Not surprisingly, this concept has profound implications for mature wellness programs.

Far too many wellness programs have been built around the premise of time telling—the hiring of an exceptionally talented and qualified person to single-handedly lead the company's wellness initiative. Unfortunately, as is all too often discovered, when the individual responsible for leading the wellness initiative burns out or decides to leave the company, the longevity of the program is jeopardized because the organization's wellness champion is gone.

Certainly, from an organizational perspective, hiring the most qualified and charismatic wellness professional available is both prudent and desirable. However, if mature programs are to increase in their stature, influence, and effectiveness—not to mention survive over time—responsibilities for corporate wellness must be disseminated to a variety of key players throughout the organization. Many additional individuals will need to be involved in the process. For example, key decision makers from such areas as occupational health, human resources, safety, management information systems, operations, and finance should be active participants in the company's wellness initiative if health promotion is expected to be successfully integrated into the fabric and culture of the company.

DEVELOPING AND COMMUNICATING ORGANIZATIONAL HEALTH INDICATORS

Whereas newer corporate wellness programs are often criticized for failing to collect data to drive their organizational health initiatives, more mature programs generally do not have this shortcoming. Indeed, most practitioners of mature programs rely on a variety of rich and meaningful data sources, including but not limited to health-risk appraisals, health screening, health care claims, absenteeism, and disability, to help them make informed decisions. When taken together, these data provide a powerful snapshot of both individual and organizational health concerns. However, given the fact that we are living in the midst of an information explosion, one must speculate whether mature programs are going to face the problem of having too much data to handle in the very near future. Indeed, living in a time when the world's information is doubling every 5 years, astute leaders of wellness programs must now concern themselves with the idea of being encumbered by too much data. As a result, a third item that demands consideration is the need for developing and communicating organizational health indicators.

Specifically, the notion of developing strategic organizational health indicators really revolves around the idea that there are four or five key pieces of data that best provide the most meaningful insight as to the true health status of the individuals within any organization. Although health promotion practitioners may be gathering and analyzing data from a multitude of sources, we believe that these data can and should be distilled down into four or five primary items.

One way to demonstrate the need for identifying key organizational health indicators is by using the illustration of the automobile dashboard. To be sure, an automobile is a complicated and intricate piece of machinery. In fact, even the most modest automobile has literally thousands of parts. Moreover, each part must work cooperatively if the automobile is to function effectively. Despite the automobile's complexity, the driver really needs to know only five or six pieces of information—the amount of gas in the tank, the speed at which it is moving, the present temperature, the oil pressure, and the number of miles since the last maintenance—to operate it. Armed with this information, which is available on the dashboard, many people who know very little about the mechanics of an automobile are able to drive with very few problems.

In the midst of an information explosion, this same thinking can and should be applied to the corporation's wellness initiative. This idea will not only force health promotion practitioners to think in terms of outcomes—what kinds of specific results should the effort and investment produce—but also will provide much needed clarity for others throughout the rest of the organization.

BROADENING OUR VIEW OF THE DETERMINANTS OF HEALTH

Practitioners of mature health promotion initiatives have traditionally concentrated their program development efforts on a relatively narrow set of individual behaviors: tobacco use, poor nutrition, sedentary lifestyles, and high-risk alcohol consumption. Because these four behaviors alone contribute to almost 50% of the nation's total annual deaths, it is not surprising to see intense organizational efforts focused on modifying these lifestyle decisions.

Although attempting to modify these kinds of unhealthy behaviors has been both an obvious and necessary place to begin, there is new and compelling research indicating that a variety of other factors may also contribute to an individual's overall sense of health and well-being (Evans, Morris, and Marmor 1994). What's more, these additional factors may even influence a person's decision to use tobacco, drink heavily, or overeat. Indeed, how employees work, what they earn, the quality and quantity of social interaction they receive throughout the course of the working day (just to mention a few) are now emerging as potential determinants of health. Ultimately, these and other related issues may provide additional insight as to why some employees are healthy and others are not. Thus, another item that deserves thoughtful consideration by the leaders of mature programs is the broadening of our understanding concerning the actual determinants of health.

Evans, Morris, and Marmor (1994) openly challenge health promotion professionals to carefully examine their beliefs about what specifically causes a person to become ill and what specifically can and should be done about it. After careful reflection, researchers are now strongly advocating that, in addition to focusing time and energy on traditional individual lifestyle behavior modification (e.g., conducting educational sessions or providing health information), health promotion practitioners should also start looking to incorporate a variety of other strategies into their action plans. Indeed, a variety of researchers now suggest that dedicating more attention to such issues as making necessary environmental modifications, designing jobs that have purpose, creating strong social support networks, balancing work and family demands, and increasing an employee's sense of purpose may all contribute to improved health and productivity outcomes.

SUMMARY

The discipline of health promotion is poised to make significant contributions to the health and well-being of the working men and women of the United States. However, the journey is not an easy one. If mature programs are to survive and thrive during this time of ambiguity and relative uncertainty, practitioners must be willing to successfully embrace the challenges that are emerging.

However, by increasing the amount of senior-level support, widening the circle to include others within the organization, developing a clear set of measurable outcomes, and embracing the ever-expanding literature that illuminates the road to better health and well-being, practitioners of mature programs will increase their likelihood of success.

REFERENCES

Chapman, L. 1997. Securing support from top management. *The Art of Health Promotion* 1:1-8.

Collins, J., and J. Porras. 1997. *Built to last: Successful habits of visionary companies.* New York, NY: HarperCollins.

Elliott, S. 1998. *Health & productivity management consortium benchmarking study: Phase II.* Ann Arbor, MI: American Productivity and Quality Center and The Medstat Group.

Evans, R., B. Morris, and T. Marmor. 1994. *Why are some people healthy and others not?* Hawthorne, NY: Aldine De Gruyter.

Heifetz, R., and D. Laurie. 1997. The work of leadership. *Harvard Business Review* 75:124-134.

Hout, T., and J. Carter. 1995. Getting it done: New roles for senior executives. *Harvard Business Review* 73:133-145.

Part III Summary

In the past, under the previous three generations of worksite health promotion, integration was viewed as a good thing to do. Now integration is vital for survival. However, accomplishing true integration and understanding all the caveats associated with it is complex. Assessment, identification, and quantification of program impact are important aspects in creating a partnership.

Mature worksite health promotion programs have a unique opportunity to form partnerships with the managed care organizations (MCOs) that provide health care coverage for their employees to enhance program outcomes. Therefore, it is proposed that measurement may in fact be an organizing principle that would allow the stakeholders (employer and MCO) to recognize how and where the program meets mutual and individual goals and objectives.

Considering the company's business interests, its social responsibilities, and the needs of its number one asset—its employees—partnerships between the worksites and MCOs around health promotion programs make good business sense.

At Dow Chemical, the cornerstone for the success of health promotion has been the development and application of the Health Promotion Management Standard. Data review led to the development of the health targets program that includes initiatives known as "Positive Action" and the "Musculoskeletal Ergonomic Strategy."

The health and productivity management model (HPM) establishes a new paradigm for working across departments and functions to put all the pieces together to form a coordinated, synergistic, and unidirectional set of solution packages. The aim of HPM is to move toward an integrated approach that is focused on people, not cases, regardless of where corporate programs reside. A synergistic team aims to coordinate care across common providers, across common conditions, across benefit plans, and across locations.

Within another model, the work promotion model, meaningful profit and meaningful employment not only coexist but also are interdependent. The employer and employee have a social contract with each other in which each side is mutually responsible for the success of the other.

Four issues are imperative when working within a mature program: increasing senior-level support, clock building versus time telling, developing key organizational health indicators, and broadening the understanding of the actual determinants of health.

Part IV

Reengineering for Mature Programs

Part Objectives

Purpose

¬ To provide readers information that will help them understand the basic concepts of reengineering and their application to worksite health promotion program development

¬ To provide readers with a visioning process that will ensure linkage of the program goals and objectives to the corporate business strategy

¬ To provide readers with a benchmarking process that will help them develop best-practice programs

¬ To provide readers several reengineering models and application examples that will help them plan appropriate utilization of reengineering tools in their programs

Application

¬ Understanding when to apply reengineering principles in health promotion programs

¬ Understanding the importance of visioning and the three-step process that can help build consensus around visioning

¬ Applying the five steps involved in benchmarking best practices that can help programs leapfrog over competition and significantly improve program outcomes and impact

¬ Understanding a reengineering process that involves institutionalizing a program into a company as an integrated component

¬ Applying a four-step organizational development model that utilizes a variety of data collection methods and analysis techniques to systematically analyze the need for program change

Vision

¬ For health promotion programs to continue to grow past program maturity, they must find and utilize a variety of tools and processes that will challenge the status quo. Reengineering efforts are one answer to the challenge of keeping program momentum alive in programs that are just a few years old. This section will force programmers to "get out of the box" and utilize techniques that will improve the creative and innovative process that many times has been lost in more mature programs.

Chapter 13

© W. Bertsch MCMLXXVI

Introducing the Concept of Reengineering

The United States Department of Health and Human Services has recognized worksites as the single most important channel to systematically provide health information and health promotion programs to adults (U.S. Department of Health and Human Services 2001). The growth of worksite health promotion programs within different work environments and among different types of employees has been impressive. The financial support literature has also grown, strongly suggesting that worksite programs have a positive impact on employee absenteeism, medical claims, and productivity (Aldana 1998). We now see many programs moving from being focused on a single risk factor to implementing multifactorial interventions offering expanded health opportunities to all employees and attracting more high-risk individuals.

Unfortunately, adding innovations and new interventions to many programs has only compounded the programs' existing problems and weaknesses. The majority of worksite programs fail to provide a systematic evaluation of their efforts and eventually become ineffective. When new interventions are added to programs that lack basic evaluation processes, program quality suffers and participation usually declines. Without a systematic evaluation process (process, impact, and outcome evaluation strategies), program improvement is almost impossible. When participation starts to drop, program administrators go into survival mode and only focus on the "low hanging fruit"—individuals and groups that are easy to reach—and they fail to gain, maintain, and grow a healthy work culture.

Many of these programs have stagnated, stopped growing, and no longer answer the challenging health needs of their work cultures. These programs have addressed few of management's health concerns or have only focused on management's needs and have failed to partner with employee groups or unions.

WHAT IS THE ANSWER?

Program administrators must recognize that problems exist and the problems presents opportunities for meaningful changes such as

¬ reengineering their programs to become the health resource that they should be;

¬ demonstrating value added to the business;

¬ partnering with other departments or employee groups and programs and increasing the ownership and program effectiveness;

¬ reaching deeper into diverse populations with more efficient services;

¬ moving stagnant programs forward;

¬ fostering an organizational culture that reinforces healthy lifestyles; and

¬ becoming a part of the business plan and not just that "wellness program."

How do you tell if your program is a good candidate for reengineering? Answer the questions in table 13.01. If you have one "yes" answer or two or more "maybes" and a "yes," your program is a good candidate for reengineering.

In the past 20 years of worksite health promotion, we have made tremendous technological strides in assessing, communicating,

Table 13.01

Reengineering Opportunity Questions

CIRCLE YOUR ANSWER TO EACH QUESTION			
The program calendar has changed very little, or there is no annual program calendar.	Maybe	Yes	No
We are doing more awareness programs than education or intervention and environment support programs.	Maybe	Yes	No
The incentive program is composed of extrinsic strategies of drawings and giveaways. It has not been tied into an ongoing company incentive program.	Maybe	Yes	No
The communication plan or elements (newsletter, flyers, posters, bulletin boards) have not been evaluated or changed, or there is no communication plan.	Maybe	Yes	No
The marketing plan has not been changed since program initiation, or there is no marketing plan.	Maybe	Yes	No
The program model fit has never been questioned, or there is no program model.	Maybe	Yes	No
The program mission, goals, objectives have not changed, or they are not in writing and have never been given to participants.	Maybe	Yes	No
Employee committees, teams, or task groups are not being used to ensure employee program ownership.	Maybe	Yes	No
It has been several years since the last satisfaction survey.	Maybe	Yes	No
It has been several years since the last employee focus group.	Maybe	Yes	No
It has been several years since the last employee needs and interest survey.	Maybe	Yes	No
It has been several years since the last management needs and interest survey.	Maybe	Yes	No
The evaluation plan has not changed or been reviewed since program initiation, or it is nonexistent.	Maybe	Yes	No
NUMBER OF MAYBE'S	**NUMBER OF YES'S**		**NUMBER OF NO'S**

and delivering health and behavior change concepts. For the first time in our field's history, employers are not questioning our worth or values. However, our program results have improved only slightly, and if we are to maintain this new era of potential growth, programs must be organized and managed to perform at higher levels of effectiveness and efficiency. New programs must be initiated using models that include best practices and processes focused on delivering results. Existing programs must be challenged to face tough questions such as those in table 13.01 and be willing to make the changes necessary to become results oriented. The twenty-first-century company that is supporting your program is demanding results.

REENGINEERING— A TRANSFORMATION PROCESS

Business process reengineering emerged as a management tool in the late 1980s. Its seeds can be found in total quality management (TQM) philosophies (Feigenbaum 1991; Atkinson 1990) and Deming's focus on quality (Deming and Juran 1991) that helped Japan rise from the ashes of World War II. Deming-style TQM was process-focused and took a holistic view of workplace activities. TQM practices were seen in the late 1970s and 1980s in Western manufacturing companies, but they faced years of Western management theory in which work was broken down into discrete tasks and given to less and less skilled employees. At the same time, another development was gathering momentum, and by the late 1970s, the information rage was the focus in many companies. The mix of

these two potential management tools had caused holy wars in many companies.

Michael Hammer, an information technology consultant, wrote an article in the *Harvard Business Review* that forcefully stated that computer hardware was not the answer to higher productivity (Hammer and Champy 1993). He suggested that Deming's focus on tightening processes and eliminating unnecessary and redundant steps was the only answer. This view gave birth to what has become known as business process reengineering and has been used by many different types of companies to improve their competitiveness and productivity.

What does business process reengineering have to do with worksite health promotion programs? Worksite health promotion programs can use the process to refocus their efforts on their clients and obtain better program results. Hammer defined reengineering as the "fundamental rethinking and radical redesign of business processes to achieve dramatic improvement" (Hammer and Champy 1993). Health promotion programs can use this same tool to become more competitive and more productive.

KEY ELEMENTS OF REENGINEERING

Three key elements have been identified in successful reengineering efforts. Figure 13.01 has been adapted from Carr and Johansson (1995) and shows the key elements relationship to other important factors.

Process Focused

What does it mean to be process focused? A process is a set of linked activities. In a health promotion program, a key process is registration. The registration process can be drawn into a process flow chart that can simply depict the tasks in an orderly sequence. The first step in

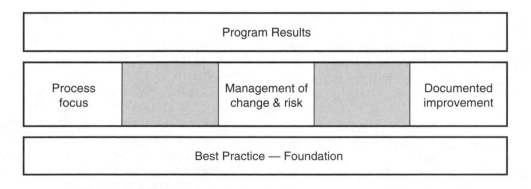

Figure 13.01 Key elements of the reengineering effort.

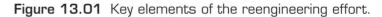

133

Table 13.02

Analysis of Health Promotion Program Registration Process

TASK	DESCRIPTION
1	Decide on a number of different ways participants will be registered (computer, registration table, registration box, mail-in registration form, and sign-up at first activity session).
2	Decide on the information that is necessary for program registration (name, demographics, and company or department information) and what information is necessary to safely and successfully administer the program and help in the final report.
3	Ensure that necessary information can be collected using different registration points.
4	Decide how information will be recorded and used in analysis of program results.
5	Put registration materials together.
6	Pilot test registration materials and fine-tune process.
7	Implement registration process.
8	Record data and use in final program analysis.
9	Evaluate registration process with staff and participants.

drawing a process flow chart for registration is to prepare an analysis of the activities as in the example in table 13.02. What tasks must be performed in the registration process? How are these tasks performed and by whom? How are the tasks sequenced, and how does the work flow? How much time is consumed during and between each task? What technologies are used during these tasks?

After you have completed a task analysis, you will draw a flow chart of the different steps. The flow chart will help you discuss the process with employees who will provide feedback about what worked and what did not work. Staff should also provide feedback about what steps took too long or which steps were unnecessary. Once you have received this feedback, you are ready to reengineer the process with ideas and suggestions from those directly involved with the process. Tightening up the processes involved in health promotion program administration not only ensures that staff is not involved in wasteful tasks but also results in higher participation rates from employees who feel less hassled by the process.

Managing Change and Risk

What does managing change and risk in a reengineering project mean? One of the reasons many health promotion programs have failed to grow is that they have become afraid of change. Bridges (1991), in his book *Managing Transitions: Making the Most of Change*, makes a bold distinction between change and transition. Change is situational. An example of change would be a new program model or a new assessment tool for cardiovascular risk factors. Transition is the psychological process that people go through to come to terms with the change.

Change is external; transition is internal. If a new program delivery system is to be successfully implemented, staff must make a fairly smooth transition to the new delivery method. Remember, change always means someone must give something up. What is being given up could look like a large risk; thus, it is important to help individuals understand and manage risk.

Following are some of the basic steps to consider when managing change and transition:

¬ Determine what individual behavior and attitude will have to be for the change to work.

¬ Analyze who stands to lose something under the new system.

¬ Effectively sell the problem so that individuals will buy into the solution.

¬ Let disgruntled clients and participants explain the problem to staff. This approach lets staff hear the problem first-hand.

¬ Talk about the difference between change and transition with staff and participants.

¬ Hold regular staff and participant meetings to discuss the progress.

¬ Always ensure an open atmosphere where staff or participants feel that they can express their opinions.

Document Improvement

The last core element of a reengineering effort is to document the improvement. This step sounds logical, but many health promotion programs are still managed by individuals who make decisions on the basis of

Table 13.03

Registration Process Table With Improvement Measures

TASK	DESCRIPTION	IMPROVEMENT MEASURES
1	Decide on number of different ways participants will be registered (computer, registration table, registration box, mail-in registration form, and sign-up at first activity session).	Document discussion for use in other registration projects
2	Decide on the information that is necessary for program registration (name, demographics, and company or department information) and what information is necessary to safely and successfully administer program and help in final report.	Document discussion for use in other registration projects
3	Ensure that necessary information can be collected using different registration points.	
4	Decide how information will be recorded and used in analysis of program results.	Document discussion for use in other registration projects
5	Put registration materials together.	
6	Pilot test registration materials and fine-tune process.	Document results
7	Implement registration process.	Count number of times each method is used
8	Record data and use in final program analysis.	Ensure ease and reliability of recording
9	Evaluate registration process with staff and participants.	Random telephone call to participants asking 3 to 5 questions concerning registration process

"gut feelings" or "experience." These programs usually have failed to collect and record the necessary information to make good business decisions. Reengineering efforts are focused on results that can be measured and documented. The key to documenting improvement is to look for the measures that can be realistically recorded and managed over the life of the process.

For example, what would be the realistic measures in documenting the improvement with our new registration system? (See table 13.03.)

BEST PRACTICES FOR REENGINEERING PROJECTS

Q In their book *Best Practices in Reengineering*, Carr and Johansson (1995) discuss with their clients 16 best practices that they have discovered. The following list is adapted from their work and the work of Bennis and Mische (1995):

¬ Gain and maintain management support.

¬ Create buy-in by articulating the need to change, and continue to communicate this need.

¬ Use a structured framework to drive the reengineering team.

¬ Create a strong link between the project goals and overall program goals.

¬ Focus on the needs or desires of the different clients (participant, employee, dependent, hard-to-reach employee, staff, and management).

¬ Do not try to reengineer too many processes at once. Prioritize your targets.

¬ Put a team of staff, employees, and management together to drive the process.

¬ Carefully choose the measures you will document for the entire process.

¬ Carefully consider the change and transitions, and put plans together to work through these steps.

SUMMARY

Reengineering is always more than just rethinking specific processes in our programs. It always involves staff, employees, and management in change. Thus, it is important that we think about the impact these changes will have on employees, staff, and management, and then plan reengineering projects using recognized best practices.

REFERENCES

Aldana, S.G. 1998. Financial impact of worksite health promotion and methodological quality of the evidence. *Art of Health Promotion* 2:1-8.

Atkinson, P.E. 1990. *Creating culture change: The key to successful total quality management.* San Diego: Pfeiffer & Company.

Bennis, W., and M. Mische. 1995. *The 21st century organization: Reinventing through reengineering.* San Francisco: Jossey-Bass Publisher.

Bridges, W. 1991. *Managing transitions: Making the most of change.* Reading, MA: Addison-Wesley.

Carr, D.K., and H.J. Johansson. 1995. *Best practices in reengineering: What works and what doesn't in the reengineering process.* New York: McGraw-Hill.

Deming, W.E., and J.M. Juran. 1991. Dueling pioneers. *Business Week* 25:17.

Feigenbaum, A.V. 1991. *Total quality control, 3rd edition.* New York: McGraw-Hill.

Hammer, M., and J. Champy. 1993. *Reengineering the corporation: A manifesto for business revolution.* New York: Harper Business.

U.S. Department of Health and Human Services. 2001. *Healthy People 2010.* McLean, VA: International Medical Publishers.

Chapter 14

Linking Reengineering to Corporate Strategy

Imagine that you've just arrived in your office on a Monday morning to begin your day. There is a message on your voice mail asking you to come to the boardroom for a special interview in 15 minutes. You enter the room and take a seat across from someone you've not seen before. The woman introduces herself as a consultant who has been hired to review your company's operations. She's holding a stopwatch. She slides a piece of paper across the table to you. On it, you read: "What is the purpose of your department? You have 30 seconds to respond."

The stopwatch begins to tick. What is your response? Do you articulate a clear sense of purpose for your department? Or does your tongue get tied in a knot trying to justify health promotion and behavior change theory and the stemming of health care cost increases?

What Language Do You Speak?

As you begin the visioning process, be sure you are using the right language and format. Although this chapter suggests some language and formats that can be useful, recognize that each organization has its own unique way of defining terms such as vision, mission, goal, objective, strategy, and tactics. To communicate your ideas clearly, you must do so in your company's native language and format your final document in a way that is familiar to its readers.

Do you walk out of the meeting (a) confident about your response or (b) concerned about what you said, or what you didn't get to say, or about who else will be asked this question?

For those who need motivation to initiate a visioning process, consider the following three reasons:

1. Vision brings business-relevant meaning to Work. We are fortunate in the field of health promotion in that it is easy to find the work of promoting health meaningful on a personal level. However, as the introductory scenario demonstrates, there must be a business-relevant meaning to your program as well.

2. Vision provides a decision platform. A strong sense of the business purpose of your department provides a basis for decision making. It should impact decisions of every magnitude, from who you should hire, to what conferences you should attend, to what journals you should receive, to whom you should take to lunch today.

3. Vision provides a stable horizon to measure progress. Like jogging or riding a bike with your view of the horizon providing instant and ongoing feedback of your progress, your vision provides a consistent sense of direction and distance for your department.

THREE-STEP VISIONING PROCESS

Table 14.01 describes a three-step process for creating and documenting a business-relevant vision for your department. The accompanying narrative provides additional insight and instruction to help you implement the process.

STEP 1: ASSEMBLE YOUR VISION TEAM AND ADVISORS

S R Your objective in this first step will be to get the right people, armed with the right information, to eagerly assist you in defining and articulating a business-relevant vision for your department. You will need two groups of people: (1) a small team that will help you do the work of developing a vision and (2) a network of advisors who will provide insightful and honest feedback regarding what you and your team create.

Visioning Team

In general, your team should comprise a facilitator and approximately six individuals that will assist in doing the bulk of the work involved in the visioning process. Roles and attributes are as follows:

¬ The facilitator is charged with objectively administering the visioning process. In meetings, the facilitator's role is to set the stage for creativity and decision making by ensuring that (1) the team has the information it needs, (2) important issues are identified and explored and finally brought to conclusion, and (3) the team makes progress toward to goal of creating and documenting their vision in a timely manner. The facilitator needs only to be experienced in leading visioning

processes; he or she does not necessarily need to have health promotion expertise.

The Player-Coach?

It is best, if possible, to have the visioning process facilitated by someone not intimately tied to its outcome. Having someone from the team as facilitator risks either (a) having that person's opinions outweigh those of the team or (b) that person suppressing his or her opinion for fear of appearing nonobjective. It's a very fine line that is difficult to walk.

¬ The team, under the direction of the facilitator, will be responsible for information collection and analysis, critical thinking, creating, and composing. The content knowledge of the team should revolve around employee health and productivity issues. Members of your department staff and representatives from such related departments as medical, safety, benefits, and human resources may all be involved.

Advisors

The role of the advisors will be to provide feedback regarding the work of your team within the context of what they understand about the broader organizational strategy. You will want six to eight advisors. In determining who your advisors should be, consider the following rules of thumb:

You will have the greatest success gaining cooperation from prospective team members and advisors if, in your approach, you do the following:

1. Clearly articulate what you are trying to do and why.
2. Define the process, timeline, and time commitment needed.
3. Be clear as to why, specifically, you are asking the individuals to help.

Table 14.01

Three-Step Visioning Process

STEP 1	STEP 2	STEP 3
Assemble vision team and advisors	Complete situation analysis (SWOT)	Develop, test, and document consensus vision

4. Make the requests in person. Don't rely on e-mail. Take time to sit down with the people you want involved.

5. Seek power. You want your advisors to be the organization's movers and shakers—the people who really understand the business and make things happen. Keep in mind that power and title are not necessarily the same thing. Focus on power.

6. Seek logical balance. Your advisors should represent a variety of perspectives, including human resources, production, labor (if applicable), and strategic planning.

7. Identify champions. You will want one or more of your advisors to be advocates of health promotion. Assuming they meet the power criteria, they will be vital to your efforts to sell the vision through the organization once it is complete.

8. Identify skeptics. You will want one or two skeptics as well. Again, if they are in power positions, you need to understand any fundamental arguments they may pose against health pro-motion activities. Often, it is the feedback from skeptics that can lead to truly breakthrough thinking, and the process itself can sometimes make them less skeptical.

STEP 2: COMPLETE SITUATION ANALYSIS

Before beginning to think about where the health promotion department is going, your team needs to understand where it is. Specifically, the goal is to define current strengths, weaknesses, opportunities, and threats (SWOT) related to health promotion in your organization.

The Information You Want

The SWOT analysis will likely be intensive and time-consuming. There are no good shortcuts to providing the perspective necessary for good visioning. Table 14.02 highlights the types of issues that should be explored with respect to the SWOT analysis of your organization's health promotion situation. Much thought should be given to what issues need to be investigated in your organization before embarking on research.

How You Get Information

In general, the information you need to identify strengths and weaknesses can be uncovered in a thorough audit of your department and all aspects of its operations. Looking at information found outside your department identifies the opportunities and threats. You may use the following tools to identify opportunities and threats:

¬ Strategic plan review. At the core of your department's business-relevant vision will be a thorough recognition of what your organization's most important goals are and what is being done to achieve them. Annual reports and Web sites reveal much of this information, but nothing can replace good questions asked of people in power.

¬ Stakeholder interviews. These interviews with key individuals inside and outside your organization can provide a knowledgeable perspective on the issues at hand. Stakeholders will likely include all of your advisors and may also include representatives from health plans or third-party administrators and others outside the organization who have insights about health and productivity issues.

¬ Data analysis. Health- and productivity-related data, such as health care claims, pharmacy records, productivity measures, and workers' compensation claims, all hold information that may reveal business-relevant opportunities for your department.

SWOT Product

When you have completed your thorough situation analysis, you should be able to compile a concise document that outlines the strengths and weaknesses of your current department, and the opportunities and threats your department faces as it looks to the future.

STEP 3: DEVELOP, TEST, AND DOCUMENT CONSENSUS VISION

This third step begins when the vision team agrees that the SWOT analysis is an accurate summary of the situation of the health promotion department. Armed with these conclusions and the data that supports them, the vision team can turn its attention

Table 14.02

Example of a Health Promotion SWOT Analysis

SWOT	SAMPLE ISSUES
Strengths	What physical assets (such as fitness centers and education facilities) are available through your department?
	What are your department's most successful programs?
	What processes and systems have been developed that consistently have successful results?
	Which relationships (internal or external) are successful?
	What are your department's specific strengths in terms of staffing and skills?
	Who are your department's supporters among the organization's leadership?
Weaknesses	What physical assets do you consistently feel are lacking?
	Where, programmatically, does your department have gaps or simply not have much success?
	What processes and systems are missing or consistently fail to produce good results?
	Where are you missing key relationships or are relationships unproductive?
	Where are there gaps in people or skills needed to succeed?
	Who are your department's detractors among the organization's leadership?
Opportunities	What are some of the critical unmet needs of your organization related to the health and productivity of employees, dependents, and retirees?
	Who else is working on health and productivity issues? Where can you work with them to achieve a common goal?
	What resources (internal or external) are not currently being used for health promotion–related activities that could be used to help your program expand or enhance its offerings?
Threats	Who else (internal or external) is working on health and productivity issues that could threaten or overtake your department's role?
	What situations (i.e., poor corporate performance) could impact your funding?
	What changes in the organization (i.e., evolution to telecommuting or greater dispersion of the workforce) could render your department's current programs and approach obsolete?

from the issue of "Where are we?" to "Where are we going?"

Format of the Vision Document

Knowing the format of what you are developing up front will make the development process much easier than proceeding blindly. The first rule to follow in formatting a vision document is to look first for internal standards. How does your organization communicate its own vision? How do other departments communicate what they see as their business purpose?

In the absence of such models, consider using a simple question-and-answer format. The following questions may serve as a template for your vision document:

¬ Why does our department exist?

¬ What distinguishes our department from other entities involved in health and productivity?

¬ What is our vision? What will the future bring if we succeed?

¬ What goals do we need to accomplish to realize this future vision?

Process of Creating the Vision Document

The work of developing a vision document will require a cycle of meetings in which your team creates and refines the vision document and visits with advisors who provide feedback on what the team has done.

¬ First vision team meeting. This meeting should be combined with review and discussion of the situation analysis so that the rationale behind the SWOT conclusions are fresh on everyone's mind. Use the second half of this meeting to create a first draft of the vision document (according to an agreed-on format). Depending on how comfortable the team is with what they create in this first draft, they may decide to meet again to refine the draft further before sharing with advisors.

¬ Share draft with advisors. Schedule face-to-face meetings with advisors. Share briefly the conclusions of the SWOT analysis and confirm understanding and agreement. Then review and discuss draft vision. The idea is to get feedback. You may need to probe for reactions. Cover issues point by point, making sure the advisor understands the meaning and implications of what is written. Compile feedback from all advisors into a summary report and distribute to vision team members before the second meeting.

¬ Second vision team meeting. The team reviews comments of the advisors. Look for contradicting opinions of advisors. Weigh all feedback, taking into consideration the perspective of the individual advisors. Use feedback to create a second draft.

¬ Repeat process to conclusion. The process of drafting, seeking advisor input, and redrafting could cycle a number of times. As the document becomes more refined, the pool of advisors who need to be briefed on subsequent revisions may shrink, depending on the issues being addressed. Likely, after two or three cycles, you will have succeeded in creating a document that clearly communicates the business purpose of your department in a manner that is acceptable to your vision team and advisors.

Stimulating Visionary Thinking

Sometimes, breakthrough, visionary thinking just happens. However, the likelihood of it just happening for everyone on your vision team at the scheduled time of your meetings is remote, so your facilitator will want to encourage visionary thinking. One useful way to stimulate visionary thinking is with an exercise in which your team takes a mental trip into the future.

The facilitator asks your team to relax, close their eyes, and imagine a typical day in the life of your organization 3 to 5 years in the future. They are asked to imagine that the health promotion department has had 3 to 5 years to do everything it thought necessary to improve employee health, productivity, and the bottom line.

With the setup complete, the facilitator asks team members to begin talking about what they observe happening around them. What do they see? What do they hear? What do they feel is happening at this future time. Ask them to place themselves in different locations, such as a remote office, the plant floor, a telecommuter's home, or a local physician's office. Again, what is happening?

While the team is responding, the facilitator records their thoughts, not stopping the flow of ideas until they stop coming, and encouraging more input if it seems the group has more to give.

At the conclusion of this exercise, the group reviews the images they have related and then turns to answering the questions or addressing the issues that drive the vision document.

Getting to Consensus

One of the most critical mistakes made in planning and vision development is a lack of attention to consensus—not confirming that those involved in the process are onboard and in support of what is being done. Such a situation must be avoided.

141

Disagreement is often a silent killer of planning processes. Because most people prefer to avoid conflict, they will not voice their disagreement—even on fundamental issues. An important job for the facilitator is to make sure everyone's opinions are represented during team meetings and among advisors by looking for and encouraging the expression of contrary opinions.

¬ Check for consensus every step of the way. Whether it is in defining the issues to investigate in the situation analysis, interpreting the analysis of the SWOT, or defining the distinctive characteristics of the health promotion department in the vision statement, you need to stop and ask if everyone agrees with what is being proposed. Consensus is particularly important in the early stages because the assumptions you will make will become the foundation of the decisions that will follow. Fundamental disagreements early in the process, if not dealt with, will bring all your work crashing to the ground later.

¬ Identify issues behind disagreements. Strong disagreements are frequently about more than the argument at hand. Often, there is a more basic difference in assumptions that needs to be dealt with. For instance, a disagreement over whether to build healthy lifestyle incentives into health plan copayments may not be about plan design but about the long-term effectiveness of external incentives.

¬ When possible, use objective data to resolve conflict over important issues. It is important to get beyond personal beliefs about what does and does not work and to look at what has happened with other organizations that have adopted similar propositions.

SUMMARY

Historically, the profession of health promotion has been on the defensive, a corporate accessory under constant threat of the budget ax. Only by defining and pursuing a business-relevant vision can health promotion professionals become more confident that their programs will not only survive but also thrive into the future.

Chapter 15

© Photri, Inc.

Benchmarking Best Practices

Benchmarking has been defined as the search for those industry best practices that lead to superior performance (Camp 1989). The definition concentrates on achieving superior performance and suggests that best practices should be pursued regardless of whether they are inside or outside the health promotion industry. The major goal of this process is to discover the secrets of success that the "best of the best" are practicing and to copy them. It should be a proactive process and approached on a partnership basis in which both parties expect to share information. This activity might sound like industrial espionage, but because benchmarking focuses on the practice and methods, discussions with competitors are not unusual and can be organized to skirt proprietary and sensitive topics.

In Arthur Andersen's book *Best Practices: Building Business with Customer-Focused Solutions* (Hiebler, Kelly, and Ketterman 1998), the authors discuss what Arthur Andersen's 50,000 employees have learned about the benchmarking process. They warn against the limited insights gained by an industry-focused approach. In an industry-focused approach, the benchmarking process becomes a game of catch-up, and it does not help companies make forward progress or move ahead of their competitors.

The authors also warn about another traditional benchmarking approach, which is to organize through the lens of function. In the health promotion industry, function might be defined by the core task areas performed by the administrative staff, health educators, personal trainers, program planners, sales people, and the other defined players in our industry. But the functional approach also limits the application of best-practice insights and narrows the potential ideas and solutions. A benchmarking process should offer the potential that the ideas and solutions gained would help you leapfrog over competitors or significantly improve your productivity.

BENCHMARK PROCESS— FIVE STEPS TO BENCHMARKING SUCCESS

Most books suggest that the best practice is to take a universal approach. This process is not limited to any specific industry, function, or geographic region. Because the universal approach is grounded in general rather than industry-specific terms, it is more flexible and readily adapted to a variety of situations. The universal approach facilitates the exchange of creative solutions and fosters the view of a common playing field on which both partners can be winners.

STEP 1—WHERE TO START

The benchmarking process starts with several questions that help define the process or processes we will benchmark:

¬ What fundamental process are you trying to improve?

¬ Are the processes rated according to your strengths and weaknesses?

¬ What stakeholders, customers, or clients do these processes effect (and you are trying to serve better)?

Benchmarking works best when you can translate fundamental processes into a key business process. This approach allows you to cast a wider net when you are looking at best practices. What would be considered a key business in a health promotion program? We could take one of the accepted health promotion models and use the primary phases or steps as key business processes.

Health Promotion Key Processes

Q The following list will provide a starting place for you to develop your own key business process list.

¬ Mission and goal setting

¬ Structure and strategy

¬ Planning

¬ Communication and marketing plan

¬ Incentive systems

¬ Program delivery systems

¬ Evaluation and reporting system

These key business processes can be divided into many subprocesses. An example would be the communications plan or strategy. Some subprocesses you might consider are material development and design, material purchase, material delivery, material evaluation, and redesign. Key business processes can be subdivided many ways, providing many different benchmarking opportunities. The more universal the process, the greater the opportunity to benchmark in a variety of industries. Additionally, the more industries, the greater opportunity to increase the number of ideas and solutions to help you be more creative and successful.

Rating Functions for Strengths and Weaknesses

After considering what functions are important for the benchmarking process, you need to rate these functions according to your strengths and weaknesses. Why is it important to understand these functions against a backdrop of strengths and weaknesses? Many companies (Bennis and Mische 1995) decide to benchmark their strongest function against the best in class, which is not the most productive approach. It is much more beneficial and effective to make major improvement in your weakest functions rather than making small improvement in your areas of strength. The rating process also gives you an opportunity to develop a better understanding of the business processes and how they relate to the issues that have brought you to the benchmarking starting line.

You will also acknowledge the stakeholders or different clients that are served or affected by these processes. Even more important, some of these individuals will become members of your benchmarking team. The team will help guide the process and ensure that it stays focused, is completed, and gets results.

STEP 2—THE TWO TEAMS

The second step is to form your benchmarking team. Mears (1995), in his book *Quality Improvement Tools & Techniques*, suggests two teams. The first team is called the "needs team" and focuses on identifying the internal and external needs relative to critical success factors or the process that will be benchmarked. They are concerned about identifying these success factors and then deciding what it takes to monitor these factors. The second team is called the "benchmarking team." They will take the critical success factors that have been identified and, as a first step, develop operational definitions for the critical indicators. Once the operational definitions have been developed, they will be the team that completes the benchmarking process.

Why two teams? The needs assessment team's output on critical success factors and measures ensures that the benchmark team does not go in the wrong direction or visit data sources without thinking through what is really necessary. It is important that the teams understand their specific roles and responsibilities and understand basic project-management and quality-improvement tools that will be used along the way. (See table 15.01.)

Table 15.01

ℚ Basic Project and Quality-Management Tools

TOOL	BRIEF DESCRIPTION
Flow chart	Understand the situation
Checklist	Finding facts
Pareto diagram	Identifying problems
Histograms	Identifying problems
Fishbone diagram	Categorize potential causes, problems, and issues; analyze what really happened
Scatter diagram	Determine relationships
Run or control charts	Compare periods and find patterns
Brainstorming	Planning; decide group's direction
Tree diagram	Map out path and task that need to be accomplished
Force field diagram	Identify obstacles to reaching goal

Adapted from Mears 1995; Chang and Niedzwiecki 1993; Baker 1998.

There are many project-management and quality-management tools that could be used to help the benchmarking teams complete the process. It is important that these groups have a facilitator that can walk the teams through the process and the use of the different tools. Without this facilitation, teams become bogged down in team administration instead of focusing on the benchmarking process.

Attributes of an Effective Team

What are the attributes of an effective team? The following list, adapted from Mears (1995), gives characteristics of an effective team.

1. The atmosphere is informal and relaxed.
2. Virtually everyone participates in the discussion and the discussion remains pertinent to the team's major task.
3. The team's task is accepted and understood by all team members.
4. Members listen to each other. Every idea is given a hearing.
5. The team is comfortable with disagreement.

6. Most decisions are reached by consensus.
7. Criticism is frequent and frank.
8. Team members are free to express their feelings and ideas.
9. Clear assignments mean action.
10. The team's chairperson does not dominate.
11. The team keeps track on how it is doing.

STEP 3—IDENTIFY PARTNERS

Partners should be chosen from outside of the health promotion field to increase the opportunity for more creative processes and results.

Benchmarking Types Affect Partnerships

There are four different types of benchmarking efforts that have been identified (Camp 1989), and each can be relevant to different program needs. The first benchmarking type is *internal operations*. It is probably the easiest for data collection. In an internal operations process, different functions, business groups, or operating units would be used as the benchmarking partners. The next potential benchmarking effort is *competitive benchmarking*. Competitors will probably be the most difficult group to pursue. It is important to ensure that size is comparable when looking at competitors. The size of an operation will usually significantly change basic functions within the operation. The third benchmarking type is a *functional benchmark leader within your industry*. These types are the best in specific functions. A good example would be the firm that has the best-in-class incentive program. The trick is to determine who is best in class for a specific function. Sources such as benchmarking organizations, consultants, industry reports, business and trade journals, and government agencies are just a few of the places you might look to get an indication about who is best in class for a function. The last benchmarking type is *best-in-class generic*. The benefit of this type is that it will uncover methods and practices that are not being used in the health promotion industry. Generic benchmarking holds the potential of revealing the "best of the best" practices.

Step 4—Collect and Analyze Data

This step begins with a discussion and agreement on what methods will be used to collect and record the information. Table 15.01 provides a list of the types of tools that can be used to collect and analyze data. Individuals who are responsible for the collection and analysis of data must become proficient in the methods that will be used.

Some of the first data that will be collected is called the baseline data. It measures and documents the flow of activities in the process that is being benchmarked. It represents both quantitative and qualitative information. The baseline data help identify and underscore the importance and value of the benchmarking activities as they relate to the vision, goals, and company direction. They also help identify goal improvement.

There are many different data-gathering approaches. Data can be collected from library databases or from internal publications and records. Data can also be collected from external data management sources, such as professional or trade associations, special industry reports, or universities, and through original research. Original research data are gathered through phone surveys, focus groups, electronic surveys, paper surveys, interviews, and site visits.

Performance Gaps

After data have been collected and analyzed, a performance gap must be determined. Performance gap is a measure that reveals the difference of your performance against the best in class. A positive gap should receive appropriate recognition, but a negative gap suggests an undesirable performance and provides the basis for improvement. It is important that gap comparisons be made with both qualitative and quantitative data. Qualitative data explain "why the metric is what it is" and provide the reason for the performance gap. Performance gap data and information collected must be analyzed in accordance with the original client or customer requirements.

Step 5—Take Action

This step could be the production of a report or a presentation based on the findings. Once the performance gap has been established, future performance levels must be established. Future performance levels are based on past history, the performance gap, and realistic future expectations. After the performance levels have been established, the benchmark finding and the new performance levels must be communicated upstream and downstream.

Critical in the communication process is gaining and obtaining acceptance. A multifaceted communications strategy will ensure that your message has an opportunity to reach deep enough within the organization to gain acceptance. What does acceptance mean? You are after acceptance from multiple layers within the organization to increase the opportunity for success of your action plan.

Once a level of acceptance has been reached that allows you to move to action planning, there are two important implementation facets to consider. The first deals with activity or task and involves defining the *who, what, when,* and *how* of the task. The second is to ask, *How will support for implementing the changes be obtained from the organization?*

The following steps have been adapted from Camp's (1989) list of task considerations and can be used to guide your action planning:

¬ The task should be specific and clear for those responsible for implementation.

¬ The steps to accomplish the task should be described in a logical order.

146

¬ The resources needed to accomplish the task should be determined.

¬ The schedule for the task should be defined.

¬ Responsibility and accountability for the task should be defined.

¬ The deliverables expected from implementation of the task should be described.

¬ Measurements from the results of implementing the task should be specified.

The last process in step 5 is to implement the actions and finally recalibrate the benchmarks.

SUMMARY

The five steps in the benchmarking process include determining where to start, forming two benchmarking teams, identifying benchmarking partners, collecting and analyzing the data, and taking action to reduce performance gaps. The benchmarking process is continuous and should be performed by those who are responsible for implementing the findings. An organization should be encouraged to take pride in benchmarking because it increases competitiveness and productivity.

REFERENCES

Baker S. 1998. *The complete idiot's guide to project management*. New York: Alpha Books.

Bennis, W., and V. Mische. 1995. *The 21st century organization: Reinventing through reengineering*. San Francisco: Jossey-Bass Publishers.

Camp, R.C. 1989. *Benchmarking: The search for industry best practices that lead to superior performance*. New York: Quality Resources.

Chang, R.Y., and M.E. Niedzwiecki. 1993. *Continuous improvement tools: Volume I & II*. Irvine, CA: Richard Chang.

Hiebler, R., T.B. Kelly, and C. Ketterman. 1998. *Best practices: Building your business with customer focused solutions, Arthur Andersen*. New York: Simon & Schuster.

Meurs, P. 1995. *Quality improvement tools & techniques*. New York: McGraw-Hill.

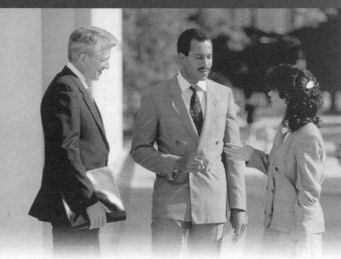

Chapter 16

© W. Bertsch MCMXC

Institutionalizing Worksite Health Promotion: Heart Check

If worksite health promotion is to reach its true potential, more creative ways are needed to take this promising concept into the business mainstream or institutionalize it. Institutionalization refers to the attainment of longevity or the final stage of innovation diffusion, in which new programs "settle" into their host organizations as integrated components (Goodman and Steckler 1989). Therefore, the purpose of this chapter is to document the efforts of one academic center to find solutions to a regional deficit in worksite activity. The results of this effort should have wider application to other areas and institutions.

THE CENTER FOR WORKSITE HEALTH

Worksite health promotion exists throughout the country, but depending on location, it can be minimal or of modest proportion in comparison to highly publicized national experiences. This circumstance is especially true in upstate New York. Companies with excellent worksite health promotion programs do exist in the region, including the Xerox Corporation, Ford Motor Company, and IBM, among others. However, the region as a whole has little in common with other, more progressive, parts of the country.

In recognition of this problem, the Center for Worksite Health, a not-for-profit academic agency affiliated with the Research Foundation of The State University of New York, was created. The center organized an ambitious work agenda to meet the growing needs for research and regional leadership in this area. Foremost on the center's agenda was the conceptualization of a strategic plan that predisposed the expansion of worksite health efforts in upstate New York. Although the center is no longer in existence, similar initiatives by other upstate organizations have continued this process.

The following discussion, much of it still hypothetical, describes the plan as currently envisioned and the progress made in its inception to date. Because this work was largely funded by New York's Healthy Heart Program, a cardiovascular disease prevention theme is evident. However, this emphasis is consistent with those of most current worksite programs (Chapman 1997). A broader health promotion focus using the same concepts is certainly possible. In fact, later sections outline how new applications of this strategy have been utilized in a managed care setting and a cancer-related health organization.

149

THE SEVEN-STEP HEART CHECK PLAN

P On the basis of the worksite experiences of the center's directors, a review of the literature, and discussions with key individuals in the industry, a seven-step intervention strategy emerged. The plan, which borrows heavily from the organizational development (Sashkin and Burke 1987; Tichy and Beckhard 1982) and the worksite health promotion literature (O'Donnell and Harris 1994; DeJoy and Wilson 1995; O'Donnell, Bishop, and Kaplan 1997; Heirich, Erfurt, and Foote 1992; Pelletier 1997), is detailed as follows.

Step 1—Evaluate and Intervene at the Organizational Level

Q Historically, worksite health promotion has focused on the individual with an array of activities directed at employees, including workshops, educational materials, and fitness centers (Ware 1982). A number of successes have occurred, yet the results have not always been promising. This almost exclusive focus on the individual is ironic because most theories and models in the health education sciences identify the environment as a critical factor in shaping behavior (Bandura 1977; Green and Kreuter 1991; Stokols 1992). Humans will behave in large part consistent with the norms, characteristics, and resources of the environments they inhabit. As a result, a growing number of experts have advocated for a more systemwide approach in health promotion delivery that includes a major emphasis on the environment (DeJoy and Southern 1993; Allen and Allen 1986; Bellingham 1990; Minkler 1989; Sorenson et al. 1995).

This paradigm shift forces a change in emphasis in program planning. The focus is away from the employee directly and on the organizational environment. Simply stated, creating healthy environments will create healthy people. Therefore, the first step in the strategic plan was to develop an organizational assessment.

Heart Check developed out of this need. Heart Check examines and quantifies a worksite's organizational structure (e.g., its policies, services, and facilities that presumably support heart health). A dichotomous scoring system is used: the company either provides the item (+1) or does not (0). An index is constructed for the overall instrument and for each of its five subscales related to heart health (smoking, nutrition, exercise, stress, and screening) and two general program supporting areas (organizational structure and administrative support).

Conceptualized as an interview with a key corporate manager, the instrument showed evidence for internal consistency and interrater reliability; content, face, and criterion validity; and test sensitivity (Golaszewski et al. 1996a; Golaszewski et al. 1996b). More recent research shows strong relationships between subsections to the total, and for several selected sub-section relationships to self-reported health behaviors (Golaszewski and Fisher 2002). A sample of Heart Check questions has been provided in appendix 14.

As a result, we are able to easily, cheaply, and accurately measure organizational support for employee heart health.

Step 2—Provide Easy Interpretation of Organizational Support Data

In the early version of Heart Check, scoring was simply defined as a percent of optimum, both by the total scale and by each subsection. For example, if a section contained 20 items and a company identified completion of five, the percent of optimum was simply 25 (5 divided by 20). In the absence of norms, this interpretation gave decision makers an estimate of what their company was doing relative to all that they could do (percent of optimum) and allowed valid comparisons among subsections even though the number of items they contained varied. Over time, this basic feedback mechanism evolved into a more sophisticated process.

Observations after repeated use revealed a hierarchy of Heart Check items. Certain items naturally preceded others in a logical pattern of program delivery. Using what is called a Q-sort process, the original project team served as raters to develop the formal Heart Check planning matrix identified in table 16.01. As noted in the table, each number corresponds to an item in Heart Check. The project team's task was to identify where each item fit within the planning stages identified along the right-hand column. All content sections of Heart Check except Organizational Foundations were treated in this manner. The following describes each section:

Table 16.01

Heart Check Health Promotion Matrix

Organizational Foundations: This section describes traditional compensation-related elements that indirectly support employee health but are not usually under the auspices of the health promotion program.

SMOKING	NUTRITION	EXERCISE	SCREENING	STRESS	ADMINISTRATIVE	IMPLEMENTATION
					5.11 6.31 6.61	1. Start-up The structural development "must do" beginning activities; no service delivery
1.11 1.41 1.51 1.12 1.13 1.14 1.15 1.18	2.11 2.12 2.13 2.14 2.15 2.16	3.1 3.33 3.34 3.35 3.37	4.11 4.13 4.61 4.12 4.13		6.81 6.10 6.11	2. Policy and environmental enhancement Easy or logical continuations at level 1; sets up service delivery
1.21 1.61 1.31 1.32 1.33 1.35 1.37	2.17 2.51 2.61 2.71 2.41 2.55 2.43 2.57 2.45 2.47	3.41 3.91 3.10 3.42 3.44 3.45	4.62 4.81 4.15 4.71 4.72 4.75 4.77	5.11 5.41 5.71 5.12 5.13 5.14 5.15	6.62 6.72 6.91 6.92 6.75	3. Basic service delivery Information, awareness building, relatively inexpensive, onsite programs
1.34 1.36 1.38 1.39	2.12 2.52 2.54 2.56 2.46 2.48	3.11 3.51 3.61 3.12 3.53 3.62 3.13 3.53 3.63 3.14 3.43 3.46	4.32 4.63 4.12 4.33 4.33 4.34 4.73 4.13 4.74 4.76 4.78	5.21 5.31 5.72 5.22 5.32 5.73 5.23 5.33 5.81 5.24 5.34 5.82 5.25 5.35 5.83 5.84	6.63 6.85 6.93	4. Advanced Service Delivery More expensive and intrusive than level 3; broadened service delivery

From A Case Study in the Potential Use of the Internet to Enhance the Growth of Worksite Health Promotion Programs, T. Golaszewski, 1997, *Guide to Health Care Resources on the Internet,* J. Hoben (Ed), Faulkner & Gray, Inc.

1. Organizational Foundations: describes compensation-related and management style characteristics that indirectly support employee health. Although these items are important to the health climate of the organization, they are not usually under the authority of the health promotion staff and are listed and scored separately. Items in this area include: the availability of health insurance, vacation time, disability coverage, and grievance procedures.

2. Startup: refers to health promotion structural development or "must do" activities that precede any service delivery. Items within this section include: the development of a wellness committee, the setting of organizational goals for employee health, the collection of needs assessment data, and the identification of a program theme and logo. *Note:* Startup only applies to the Administrative Support section.

3. Policy/Environment Enhancement: includes easy and/or logical continuations of activity found in the above section. Items in this area lay the foundation for future service delivery, and are not particularly expensive or time demanding to initiate. Activities here include the presence of no-smoking policies and healthy vending machine food options.

4. Basic Service Delivery: provides for basic educational or service programs, such as a blood pressure screen. Elementary program elements that support these efforts, such as a promotional campaign, are also included here.

5. Advanced Service Delivery: continues the activities found in the above but broadens and enhances the degree of services provided. Generally, program elements that add to their costs and/or complexity are found in this section and include such components as providing offsite as opposed to onsite programs, using more than one form of delivery (self-study guides, software-based programs, etc.), or conducting efforts on company time.

6. Institutionalization: provides activities that lead to long-term cultural change and have significant policy or cost implications. Items in this area are not likely to be eliminated easily. As a result, they become part of the business "mainstream" (becoming institutionalized). Examples of items include: benefits enhancements for health criteria (e.g., "wellness days" off), hiring of a professional to manage program activity, and the development of a fitness center.

As currently used, a company's profile is determined by simply highlighting items that were achieved, thus providing a visual representation of its support for heart health. Using this visual pattern (the highlighted matrix), along with percents of achievement scores for each column and row, shows program directors where deficiencies occur and where likely "next step" activities should follow. For example, many companies provide health promotion services or establish a fitness center without incorporating the preliminary steps identified under start-up (e.g., conducting a needs assessment, developing a Wellness Committee, identifying program objectives). This deficit would show on the matrix and presumably prompt action to "back fill."

The conceptualization of Heart Check and the matrix add a significant component to the organizational measurement process. First, the availability of Heart check data brings quantification to a construct (organizational support) that has been largely ignored in the health promotion planning process. With a baseline score, companies can now define quantitative objectives (e.g., improve Heart Check by 20% after one year). This fundamental management practice could not have been achieved in the past. Second, with the development of the matrix and its hierarchy of program components, planning can proceed along a logical progression. These capabilities shift worksite health promotion from a disconnected series of random activities to a more coordinated and systematically-planned process.

As a result of the above, we can easily interpret and utilize organizational support data.

STEP 3—DEFINE HEART CHECK CRITERIA OF EXCELLENCE

Q Do high–health support companies provide lower risk and cost to employers than their low–health support counterparts? A compelling theoretical argument can be made that high organizational support would translate into lower employee health risks and consequently lower health care costs. Therefore, knowing the right combination of variables that define a "healthy company" would have an enormous impact on stimulating worksite health activity and potentially better managing costs.

In the absence of definitive research that defines a healthy company, alternate strategies were needed to be developed. The former New York State Wellness Works project (a spin-off of the Healthy Heart initiative) attempted such definitions. Rather than solely trying to improve Heart Check scores as a project goal, Wellness Works determined targets, or in other words, a subset of the instrument's items that were believed to comprise a healthy organization.

Two levels, defined by expert opinion, were identified for this purpose. The first level is called "heart friendly." A heart friendly company meets a collection of Heart Check criteria that supports any health initiative (e.g., presence of a wellness committee, completion of a needs assessment, identification of program objectives) and provides some basic policy changes (e.g., no smoking) and primary services (e.g., smoking-cessation programs, screenings). The criteria were chosen because they are not costly or logistically difficult to achieve and could be completed in 1 year or less. Presumably, these items working in synergy would create a company with a moderate probability of having employees at low risk of cardiovascular disease.

In contrast, a heart healthy company meets all of the heart friendly criteria, plus provides a much broader array of services and has more expensive and permanent program components. A heart healthy company, as the name implies, has taken serious initiatives to improve the health and well-being of its employees—it has institutionalized health promotion. In contrast to a heart friendly company, a heart healthy company is believed to have a high probability of having low risks of cardiovascular disease among its employees relative to comparable organizations.

STEP 4—LINK ORGANIZATIONAL STANDARDS OF EXCELLENCE TO DESIRABLE OUTCOMES

One major factor undermining health promotion's growth in small and midsized firms in particular is the lack of tangible financial benefits provided to sponsoring agencies. This statement may seem contradictory, given the growing research on the subject. However, few companies have the resources to conduct rigorous evaluation studies. As a result, most employers are left to make health promotion decisions on faith—the belief that financial gains realized in other and often very dissimilar organizations will be evident in theirs—regardless of the quality and quantity of research observed in the literature.

Ideally, this research inadequacy could be circumvented if insurers provided discounts to health promoting companies—a position advocated by the Worksite Health Alliance during the Clinton health care reform plan (Witmer 1994). Although the 1996 Health Insurance Portability Act allows modified community rating for health promoting organizations—and thus premium discounts—no insurers are known to offer this arrangement on a systematic basis. Yet, employers need to feel they are receiving tangible financial gains (insurance discounts or identifiable gains) for their investment in worksite health promotion.

Wellness Works considered recognizing companies meeting standards (heart friendly or heart healthy) through some type of citation from the United States Department of Public Health. Although it was never completed, this simple act would have allowed recognized companies to take whatever public relations advantage they could from their designation. This discussion is clearly theoretical, but it represents the direction that worksite health promotion needs to take to be considered a serious organizational pursuit—link tangible rewards to organizations of excellence.

As a result, a vision exists to link company health promotion initiatives to financially relevant outcomes.

STEP 5—DEVELOP COST-EFFECTIVE MEANS TO FACILITATE COMPANY HEART CHECK IMPROVEMENTS

Presumably, if widespread Heart Check evaluations were made, most companies would score poorly. Yet a number of organizations would probably be interested in improving, especially if some tangible rewards were linked to reaching levels of excellence (step 4). However, making sweeping improvements on organizational support for health is not easy. The Healthy Heart initiative has begun to address this concern.

Recent research indicated that providing health promotion training to mostly human resource managers from targeted companies can cost-effectively improve Heart Check scores (Golaszewski, Barr, and Cochran 1998). Using a partnership consisting of a college, a managed care company, and the state health department, a training program called the Worksite Health Promotion Seminar Series was introduced to 10 employers, simultaneously. Over the course of 10 months, company managers met for seven sessions to learn the process of planning, promoting, delivering, and evaluating worksite health promotion initiatives.

After 1 year, post–Heart Check evaluation scores increased by over 400% and were significantly greater than those observed in a group of matched comparison companies. In fact, the average organizational score for the intervention group virtually equaled those measured by Heart Check in companies serviced by one of the nation's most acclaimed worksite health promotion commercial providers (Breslow et al. 1990).

The Working Well Program offers another model of intervention. Unlike Worksite Health Promotion Seminar Series, it was delivered more widely and at a lower cost. For example, four, one-time-only training sessions, each with 20 client companies attending, were held throughout New York. At each session, previously collected Heart Check data were fed back to participants along with comparisons to heart healthy and heart friendly criteria.

Project goals were set to increase Heart Check scores by at least 20 points and to have at least 25% of participating companies reach heart friendly status after 1 year. To obtain these goals, company representatives were given a "pathway to success" action plan (driven by Heart Check criteria), with supplemental resources that were similar to those given at the seminar series. Follow-up support was provided by pairing each company representative with a "buddy" from another participating company and by regular communications from the project staff.

The goals of Working Well were less ambitious than those of the seminar series. Yet, small changes in many more companies may prove more cost-effective than those seen in the more resource intensive and selected seminar series. This project has not been evaluated, but it represents a model to provide widespread improvements on organizational support using a relatively modest investment.

The above represent two approaches used by the author to increase heart check scores and ultimately, support for employee health behavior. Many other alternatives are certainly possible and valid. For example, the overall Healthy Heart initiative in New York has funded multiple studies that have consistently showed success, regardless of the sponsoring institution or intervention approach used. In fact, in approximately 50 project trials, pre-to-post total Heart Check scores have increased on average 75%, with corresponding changes in subsection scores, such as 114% for nutrition, 143% for physical activity, and 109% for administrative support observed (Golaszewski and Fisher 2002).

As a result, we know organizational support for employee heart health can be inexpensively and efficiently improved across an entire state.

STEP 6—MONITOR WORKSHEET HEALTH PROMOTION ACTIVITY THROUGH REGULAR HEART CHECK ASSESSMENTS

Consider what would happen if wide-scale testing with Heart Check were commonplace. Such assessments would likely reveal the relatively low support that most employers provide. In New York, for example, early Healthy Heart Program research indicated a level of only 23% of Heart Check criteria met (Fisher, Golaszewski, and Barr 1999).

Experiences gained from the seminar series indicate that low scores have considerable impact on organizational decision making. When company deficits are highlighted, serious policy making for improvement often follows. By adding the dimension of continued follow-up, a measure of accountability for future outcomes is provided.

As a result, both the level of awareness for deficits in organizational support for employee health and prompts for continued action can be improved through repeated assessments.

STEP 7—ESTABLISH HEART CHECK NORMS BY INDUSTRY SIZE AND TYPE

With a mechanism to monitor Heart Check criteria in place (step 6), a substantial database can be developed. With the emergence of such a database, norms by industry type, organizational size, and public and private sector employers could easily be defined.

Strategically using this information would presumably have a motivating effect on organizational leaders and persuade them to offer more health promotion services. For example, knowing that one's company scores only 10% on a Heart Check criteria would probably stimulate some additional support for health promotion. But knowing that this score ranks the company in the bottom quartile of all comparable employers might generate even greater organizational attention (especially if one's competitors were publicizing their better scores).

The beginnings of such norms have already begun. At this point, 1,000 New York employers have been measured with Heart Check. Although the data have not been broken out by size of type of employer, standardization of results provides insights into the distribution of Heart Check criteria. For example, using known standard deviations and quartile breakdowns, and applying arbitrary labels, total Heart Check scores have assumed the following distribution: > 40% excellent; > 22%-40% good; > 15%-22% above average; 11%-15% below average; and < 11% poor (Golaszewski 2002).

As a result, the potential to grade work organizations and stimulate employer competition for status, "bragging rights," and possibly tangible rewards (see item 4), exists.

SUMMARY

A seven-step model has been proposed that takes a systemwide approach to improving organizational support for employee heart health (or any health focus for that matter). The model moves through a progression of strategies, starting with measuring organizational support, and then proceeds through stages of providing easily interpreted data for company decision makers, developing organizational targets of excellence, linking financially relevant outcomes to these targets, measuring the construct on a regional scale, and finally, developing regionwide normative standards. Work on the model has shown evidence for success, and ongoing research and innovation should offer further insights into its effectiveness.

Some of these advances have already begun. For example, Heart Check has evolved into two different models that measure employer support beyond heart health (Golaszewski, Barr & Pronk 2003). The managed care company, HealthPartners of Minneapolis, MN, has created WorkCheck, a 350-item organizational assessment that measures such additional factors as safety, maternal health, substance abuse, and workplace violence. The American Cancer Society—Eastern Division, has created Working Well, a 250-item inventory that measures support for the three major chronic diseases found in most work organizations: cancer, heart disease, and diabetes. Both of these models are undergoing pilot testing and no evaluation effects are known at this writing. Yet their existence speaks well for the growing utility that such measurement systems offer.

Additionally, legislation has been discussed in New York to allow experience-rated insurance pricing and thus, premium discounts for companies showing healthy profiles—a potential use for Heart Check or other similar tools (New York State Assembly 2001). The risk rating of companies is closer to becoming reality.

Finally, discussions have involved the use of computer technology to collect and report data on a grand scale, making this paper-based system easier to use and further stimulating the process of organizational change. With a computer-based data collection and reporting system, the use of the internet for this purpose would not be too far behind.

In conclusion, while still under development, a model exists to institutionalize the process of worksite health promotion on a regional basis and move this promising initiative into the mainstream of business activity.

REFERENCES

Allen, J., and R. Allen. 1986. From short-term compliance to long-term freedom: Culture based health promotion by health professionals. *American Journal of Health Promotion* 1:39-47.

Bandura, A. 1977. *Social learning theory*. Englewood Cliffs, NJ: Prentice Hall.

Bellingham, R. 1990. Debunking the myth of individual health promotion. *Occupational Medicine: State of the Art Review* 5:665-675.

Breslow L., J. Fielding, A.A. Herrman, and C.S. Wilbur. 1990. Worksite health promotion: Its evolution and the Johnson & Johnson experience. *Preventive Medicine* 19:13-21.

Chapman, L. 1997. Benchmarking best practices in workplace health promotion. *The Art of Health Promotion* 1:1-8.

DeJoy, D., and D. Southern. 1993. An integrative perspective on worksite health promotion. *Journal of Occupational Medicine* 35:1221-1230.

DeJoy, D., and M. Wilson (Eds.). 1995. *Critical issues in worksite health promotion.* Boston, MA: Allyn & Bacon.

Fisher, B., T. Golaszewski, and D. Barr. 1999. Measuring worksite resources for employee heart health. *American Journal of Health Promotion* 13:325-332.

Golaszewski, T., D. Barr, C. Blodgett, and R. Delprino. 1996a. Continued development of an organizational health assessment. *Worksite Health* 2:32-35.

Golaszewski, T., D. Barr, and S. Cochran. 1998. An organization-based intervention to improve support for employee heart health. *American Journal of Health Promotion* 13:26-35.

Golaszewski, T., D. Barr, and N. Pronk. 2003. The development of assessment tools to measure organizational support for employee health. *American Journal of Health Behavior.*

Golaszewski, T., C. Blodgett, D. Barr, and R. Delprino. 1996b. The development and preliminary testing of an organizational heart health support assessment. *Journal of Health Education* 27:25-29.

Goodman, R., and A. Steckler. 1989. A model for the institutionalization of health promotion programs. *Family and Community Health* 11:63-78.

Green, L., and M. Kreuter. 1991. *Health promotion planning: An educational and environmental approach, 2nd edition.* Palo Alto, CA: Mayfield Publishing Company.

Heirich, M., J. Erfurt, and A. Foote. 1992. The core technology of worksite wellness. *Journal of Occupational Medicine* 34:627-637.

Minkler, M. 1989. Health education, health promotion, and the open society: An historical prospective. *Health Education Quarterly* 16:19.

New York State Assembly, Committee on Insurance. 2001. Bill text—A05851. Albany, NY.

O'Donnell, M., and J. Harris. 1994. *Health Promotion in the Workplace, 2nd edition.* Albany, NY: Delmar.

O'Donnell, M.P., C.A. Bishop, and D.L. Kaplan. 1997. Benchmarking best practices in workplace health promotion. *The Art of Health Promotion* 1:1-8.

Pelletier, K.R. 1997. Clinical and cost outcomes of multifactorial, cardiovascular risk management interventions in worksites: A comprehensive review and analysis. *Journal of Environmental Medicine* 12:1154-1169.

Sashkin, M., and W. Burke. 1987. Organizational development in the 1980s. *Journal of Management* 13:393-417.

Sorenson, G., J.S. Himmelstein, M.D. Hunt, R. Youngstrom, and J.K. Ockene. 1995. A model worksite cancer prevention: Integration of health protection and health promotion in the Well Works Project. *American Journal of Health Promotion* 10:55-62.

Stokols, D. 1992. Establishing and maintaining healthy environments: Toward a social ecology of health promotion. *American Psychologist* 47:6-22.

Tichy, N., and R. Beckhard. 1982. Organizational development for health care organizations. In *Organizational development in health care organizations*, ed. N. Margulis and J. Adams, 10-20. Reading, MA: Addison-Wesley.

Ware, B. 1982. Health education in occupational settings; history has a message. *Health Education Quarterly* 9(suppl):37-41.

Witmer, R.W. 1994. Worksite health promotion and health care reform: An update. *American Journal of Health Promotion* 9:5-8.

Chapter 17

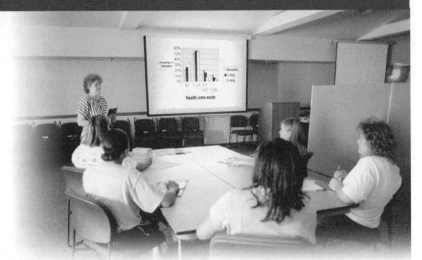

Promoting Reengineering With the Organizational Development Model

Why do companies or departments seek organizational development (OD) solutions to improving performance or competitiveness? An organization is much like an individual who has various systems working inside in varying states of health. When an individual is unhealthy, various warning signs will appear and the individual will take steps to assess and fix the problems.

The purpose of OD is to keep organizations as healthy and efficient as possible. Companies will utilize OD approaches in the following circumstances:

¬ Key individuals cannot get along.

¬ People are unfocused and unclear about their personal and professional goals.

¬ Teams are performing poorly, fighting with each other, or both.

¬ Quality is poor, customer service is bad, turnover is high, complaints are up, and employee morale is down.

¬ The organization is out of touch with its clients and customers.

OD focuses on performance and process values that empower employees, create open communication systems, promote culture collaboration and continuous learning, and facilitate the ownership of process and outcome

(Ralphs 1996). The following circumstances in a health promotion department provide the potential for an OD solution:

¬ The opportunity to reengineer programs into the health resource they should be

¬ Opportunities to demonstrate value added to the business

¬ Opportunities to partner with other departments or employee groups or programs and increase the ownership and program effectiveness

¬ Opportunities to reach deeper into diverse populations with more efficient programs

¬ An opportunity to move stagnant programs forward

¬ Opportunities to foster an organizational culture that reinforces healthy lifestyles

¬ Opportunities to become a part of the business plan and not just that "wellness program."

These types of opportunities offer increased potential of success for an OD process. This type of work is generally completed with the help of an OD consultant or in-house OD specialists. Because this approach sets up a highly interactive relationship between the consultant or specialists and the program team, the degree of "ownership" and collaboration is one of its major assets. This approach makes the OD process very different from other processes that require the help of internal or external consultants, who focus only on benchmarking, problem solving, or development of a new intervention without program staff help.

Reengineering, as an OD tool and process unlike continuous improvement and benchmarking, is intended to quickly and drastically change a system or process (Tenner and De Toro 1997). Instead of incremental changes and gains that might be planned in a continuous improvement process, reengineering planning is focused on rapidly achieving new performance levels. Thus, reengineering requires determination and commitment from both the health promotion team and management. Many programs will find that reengineering is not the appropriate approach because of the inability of the program staff or management to make the commitment necessary for the project to be successful.

Note: Before a reengineering project can be started, the mandate for change must come from the stakeholders, and the organization's readiness for change must be apparent. Without these two conditions, reengineering efforts are doomed to failure.

BASICS OF THE ORGANIZATIONAL MODEL

OD is generally broken down into three stages: diagnostic, planned change, and intervention (Ralphs 1996).

DIAGNOSTIC STAGE

The purpose of the diagnostic stage is to identify the problem or opportunity. It starts with a data collection and analysis step and concludes with a data feedback step. During the data collection and analysis step, gaps are identified between where the program is currently and where it would like to be in the future. During the last step, the client or stakeholder team is provided with the feedback on these gaps in a face-to-face meeting. This meeting helps develop ownership of the findings and, if structured properly, increases the motivation for moving the process forward. Once the data have been reported, there should also be a better sense of the pockets of resistance and acceptance by stakeholder groups. The most important purpose of this meeting is to lay the groundwork for the next steps of planned change and intervention.

PLANNED CHANGE STAGE

The planned change stage is organized around the gaps that have been identified in the data collection and analysis stage. Many program administrators collect and analyze data that suggest a change is necessary. They act on that suggestion by borrowing an intervention or program development tool they have read about in a trade journal or received from another program director. The change fails because of the lack of a customized intervention that truly fits their program or corporate culture and the lack of sufficient planning. This intermediary stage provides the program development team and stakeholder group an opportunity to determine the number of changes necessary to move the program forward. The following questions should be considered regarding program changes:

¬ Do they need to focus on overcoming resistance to the program?

¬ Do they need to break into or create new market segments to increase participation?

¬ Do they need to make the current program offerings more efficient to meet a budget deficit or decrease?

The number of changes that could be accomplished is varied and should be reviewed and planned for in the planned change stage if the intervention stage is to be successful. Change leaders and change agents are also identified during the planned change stage to increase the potential acceptance of the intervention. Much of their work will be in building support by converting an issue into a "felt need" for the various levels within the organization. After the intervention, the change leaders and agents will ensure that the change is ingrained into the system until it becomes the norm or a culture value for the corporation.

INTERVENTION STAGE

The intervention stage is where a variety of tools and processes are used to close the gaps that have been documented. These gaps could exist in individual, group, or organizational program issues, processes, or policies. A good example would be when the

University of Texas M.D. Anderson Cancer Center formed an Executive Excellent Group to work on their sidewalk smoking challenge. Like many hospitals, M.D. Anderson is a hospital that has a no-smoking policy but has not taken the steps to enforce the policy outside its doors. When individuals leave the buildings, they must walk through smokers and sidewalks littered with cigarette butts. The attempt to change this situation has caused angry confrontations with patients, visitors, and employee smokers. This situation is a good opportunity to utilize several OD interventions to develop a solution for the sidewalk smoking problem. At the same time, a realistic smoking-cessation strategy could also be developed to give patients, visitors, and employees a menu of ways to stop smoking. The intervention stage is focused on closing the gaps with a variety of OD tools.

REENGINEERING APPROACHES

Approaches to a reengineering challenge can follow several routes. There are many anecdotes in the health promotion literature of program directors who "just did it," saving thousand of dollars or increasing participation and compliance rates. However, these are the exceptions, and generally a high rate of failure can be expected with the "just do it" route. The lack of planning and organizational support from these efforts can be seen through the demise of program directors and their programs.

Since the mid-1980s, there has been a breed of health promotion professionals who have become worksite health promotion management and program consultants. Many of these individuals served for years as program managers and accumulated the experience and knowledge necessary to help others. This second approach to reengineering can be expensive, but it also offers a way to meet an urgent need for change. When a program relies 100% on a consultant they eliminate the opportunity for organizational learning and the need for the organization to develop its own expertise is eliminated. Unfortunately, the success of subsequent reengineering projects is probably low unless the same consultant is utilized again.

The last route is for the organization to understand the need for change and decide to build its own internal capabilities with the help of a consultant. Consultants might be hired to help reengineer changes, but they are also expected to help build the internal process and capabilities that could be used in future change projects. Although this approach might sound like a more difficult path, it becomes easier as experience is built. The process that follows utilizes this last route and has been applied successfully to large and small worksite health promotion change projects in a variety of industries.

A partial list of industries and clients where this model has been applied includes the following:

Energy Companies

¬ Chevron USA—application of the model to look for behavior change barriers

¬ PSE&G—application of the model reinitiated their program with broader support

¬ Tenneco—used to move an internationally recognized fitness center based program into a model that serviced employees with and without fitness centers and was recognized by American Productivity & Quality Center for "Program Excellence" after application of the model

¬ Reliant Energy—model helped refocus evaluation efforts:

Government

¬ Royal Canadian Mounted Police— model was taught to 18 health educators who serviced the RCMP groups throughout Canada:

Hospital & Pharmaceutical

¬ Johns Hopkins Hospital & Health System—recognized by AWHP as Outstanding Hospital Program after the model was applied.

¬ Pfizer Pharmaceutical—won a C. Everett Koop Award after the model was applied

¬ The University of Texas M.D. Anderson Cancer Center—reinitiated program startup following the application of the model and program review:

Service Industry

¬ Marriott International—application of the model helped move the program forward under worklife program structure

BAUN HEALTH PROMOTION REENGINEERING PROJECT MODEL

One of the challenges in developing a reengineering model that can be used successfully in worksite health promotion programs is building a process that links the practice of organizational development and health intervention modeling. There are many organizational models found in the literature (Bray 1994) that provide a representation, metaphorically, of an organization. These models are used in OD work to help categorize data about the organization, which can help enhance understanding of the weakness or opportunities. They provide a common shorthand language of terms that increase the communication efficiency among organization members. This ease of communication can lead to more effective data interpretation, which then can be linked to specific change plans. In comparison, a model in the health literature is a subclass of theory and could be built on one or several different health theories (McKenzie and Smeltzer 1997). Health models provide the framework for program directors to develop appropriate interventions. The model presented in figure 17.01 blends OD and health intervention models into four steps.

STEP 1: PROJECT INITIATION

The first step is project initiation, and during this step, the ownership of and commitment to the project is determined. The potential for a reengineering project arises when an issue or problem exists that will take a rather large or drastic change in direction. This type of change could be recognized by the health promotion program director, by management, or by the program committee. It is important to identify the value or worth of the change early in the process if it occurred.

For example, the Tenneco program started as a fitness center but, because of the level of participant interest and growth, found that it could not adequately meet the health promotion needs with the current number of staff. The program director is considering dividing the program into a fitness program and a health promotion program that would function separately but plan and coordinate offerings together. Management was interested in the proposal, but needed to see the real worth or value of this change. What might be the worth or value of this change? This change would allow the full development of staff interested in health promotion to move away from a fitness facility. It would allow the fitness staff more time to concentrate on facility updating and upkeep. However, the largest value would be gained in reaching individuals who cannot or will not use the fitness center through a more proactive health promotion program.

The program director and staff begin looking at the cost of the change and what resources

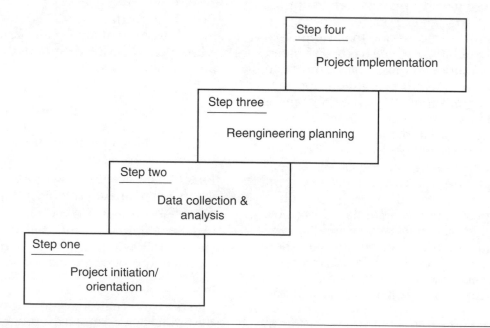

Figure 17.01 Baun health promotion reengineering project model.

would have to be channeled in other directions. They also considered what should be the goals of the proposed change project and how these goals would be measured. These issues must be answered in all programs as the process moves forward.

Once a potential project has been identified and the value of the project is understood, two teams are formed to help move the project forward. The first team formed is the project team, and it is made up of individuals who will be responsible for collecting and analyzing the data, planning the details of the reengineering project, and making the report. Some of these team members will become members of the teams that will be involved in implementing the change process. What makes a good project team member? Project team members should

¬ have specific knowled1ge of the processes that will be analyzed;

¬ understand the need for a change that will bring a new vision, direction, and position;

¬ be creative and innovative;

¬ be able to assimilate new ideas, responsibilities, and roles quickly;

¬ enjoy the challenge of change;

¬ have high energy that they can transfer to others; and

¬ be able to contribute under pressure and willing to challenge and break the necessary barriers.

The process owner team is made up of individuals who are either stakeholders or represent stakeholder groups. Svendsen (1998) defines stakeholders as individuals or groups who can affect or who are affected by the corporation's activities. In a worksite health promotion program, stakeholders can be participants, nonparticipants, managers and supervisors who run departments that provide support to the program or are supported by the program, and external individuals or groups that either support or are supported by the program. The process owner team will guide the process forward and have the responsibility to ensure that it stays on track and continues to move forward. At Marriott, the process team was the Wellness Council that was made up of a mix of senior level employees and at PSE&G the

process team was a newly formed group of individuals representing departments that had a stake in wellness. Like the two teams that were formed in the benchmarking process, these teams serve different functions that increase the opportunity for project completion and success.

Early in the project initiation step, representatives from both teams should hold a series of meetings that focus on defining the goals and objectives of the project. The goals and objectives for the process should come from the best-in-class industry standards as indicated by any of the following health promotion benchmark industry awards:

¬ AWHP Business and Industry Awards

¬ WELCOA Workplace Awards

¬ C. Everett Koop National Health Awards

¬ Fitness Management NOVA Awards

¬ APQC Benchmark Health Promotion Awards

Because of the complexity of this process, setting standards is a good task for a health promotion consultant who specializes in benchmarking. The end result of this work should be a presentation to both the project and the process owner teams that will provide them the information necessary to understand the need for and importance of intervention. It will also help them realistically match program goals to measurable outcomes. Only the stakeholders can ensure that program goals are matched to measurable outcomes because they own the data and, in many instances, the reporting processes.

Once the project goals and objectives have been identified, the data management processes must be reviewed to ensure maximization of data aggregation needs and minimization of the time necessary to make the data useable. The final phase of the initiation step is to develop a preliminary outline of the final report. This outline will ensure that the data necessary to complete the final report are collected, analyzed, and in a form the stakeholders will understand.

The Baun health promotion reengineering project model borrows from both the organizational development and health literature to create a model that can be effectively applied to worksite programs. What is unique about this model is the core focus of developing the processes and tools necessary for an internal team to effectively handle change projects. The flexibility of the model has been tested and proven many times and allows an internal team to effectively tailor the steps so that the model can be used in projects that vary in scope, purpose, and expected outcome.

STEP 2: DATA COLLECTION AND ANALYSIS

During the data collection step, the project team will choose an appropriate methodology to collect the necessary data within the established budget and time frame. Many different types of data gathering techniques can and should be utilized to increase the type and volume of data. Many organizational development project teams utilize models to guide the collection process. Bray (1994) suggests that organizational models can be useful in the following ways:

¬ Categorizing data

¬ Enhancing the OD and project teams' understanding of the data

¬ Interpreting data

¬ Providing a greater efficiency in communication relative to key terms

Health Promotion Data Collection Model

The data collection matrix presented in table 17.01 is based on the Hornstein and Tichy (1973) Technical, Political, Cultural (TPC) Matrix, and it has been specifically designed for worksite health promotion programs and applied to small and large projects. Seven key processes have been identified as best-practice components:

¬ Mission, goals, and objectives

¬ Infrastructure and strategy

¬ Planning

¬ Marketing and communications

¬ Incentive systems

¬ Program delivery and interventions

¬ Evaluation and reporting

What makes this matrix unique is that the seven processes are evaluated over three different core categories that focus on program elements that are important to program success: technical, political, and cultural.

The technical category focuses on quality, effectiveness, and efficiency issues. The political category focuses on program alignment and senior management support. The cultural category focuses on the people issues and provides a feel for the program's climate and ownership relative to health.

Data Collection Methods

Five data collection processes are employed to maximize the potential breadth of the data collected and increase the credibility of the findings. These five methods provide a cost-effective approach to collecting the vast array of data necessary to successfully implement a reengineering project.

¬ Observation. Observing committee meetings, program and intervention offerings, and group activities will allow the project team or consultant to quickly become familiar with the program and the major issues that create barriers to success. At Pfizer, observation was used during fitness and physical therapy consultations and helped uncover natural linkages that had not been utilized.

¬ Interviews. Key interviews should be conducted with different stakeholders, staff members, core participants, and employees who are either low users or represent the hard-to-reach employee. The observations will raise a set of common questions that can be used to guide the interview process, but a good interviewer will listen more than ask questions. Both the observations and the interviews will provide data that will help form the basis for focus groups. At the University of Texas M.D. Anderson Cancer Center several moths of interviewing employees at all levels of the organization helped provide management with a clear picture of the need for a better structured wellness program.

¬ Focus groups. These groups allow data to be collected quickly and provide an in-depth discussion of important

Table 17.01

Data Collection Matrix for Health Promotion Programs

KEY PROCESSES	TECHNICAL CATEGORY	POLITICAL CATEGORY	CULTURAL CATEGORY
Mission, goals, objectives	X	X	X
Infrastructure and strategy	X	X	X
Planning	X	X	X
Marketing and communications	X	X	X
Incentive systems	X	X	X
Program delivery and interventions	X	X	X
Evaluation and reporting	X	X	X

issues..Holding several focus groups that represent different participant types allows data to be categorized relative to who the participants are within the group or company. Focus groups provide a structured environment that is managed by a facilitator who asks a set of predetermined questions. Focus groups were used at Chevron USA to help clarify the behavior change barriers that employees were facing. The results of the focus groups suggested that employees did not understand readiness or stage of change. Usually facilitators do not serve as their own recorders. The person who serves as recorder should be familiar with the issues being discussed and familiar with the group of participants.

The primary source of data from the focus group should be the recorder. The secondary, or backup, source can be a tape recorder. Before the session begins, the facilitator should inform the group that he or she would like to tape the session but that the tape will not be heard by the sponsoring group. This assurance is necessary so that the participants feel they can openly discuss the topics without fear of reprisals. It is best to bring in an outsider to facilitate these sessions because the higher comfort levels among participants results in increased responsiveness.

¬ Survey. The focus group data will be utilized to develop a survey that targets the major issues that have been raised in the observations and interviews and now confirmed by the focus group. The survey is tailored to answer the tough questions. A generic survey might offer standardized validity and credibility, but the tailored survey allows you to collect the hard-to-get information. A randomized group comparison maximizes the potential survey response. Different employee participant groups (high program users, medium program users, low program users, and no program users) are given the survey, and within each group, survey participants are further stratified by demographic variables (e.g., age, gender, and job position). The survey will add breadth to the data already collected. At Marriott, where there was not a fitness center, the systems department helped ensure that the survey was sent to a randomized group that fairly represented the employee population. This data was crucial in looking for ways to help the program grow.

¬ Historical program data. This data collection method not only provides a clear picture of the current data collection and reporting process but also can be used as a backdrop against which to compare other data points. Monthly reports, annual reports, special reports, daily data runs, annual calendars, satisfaction surveys, and need and interest surveys are all part of the historical data that should be collected, reviewed, and summarized. The programs at PSE&G, Johns Hopkins, Marriott, and Reliant all had significant historical data that was used to better understand the roots of the program. Without this historical understanding, solutions can be put into place that will fail because of "fit" problems.

Application of the Data Collection Matrix

To apply the data collection matrix, a series of questions can be developed for each of the key processes within each of the three core categories of program elements. Examples of the types of questions that should be developed follow.

Program Mission, Goals, and Objectives

Technical Questions

¬ Is there a written mission statement? Are there written program goals? Are there written program objectives to support the goals?

¬ Have the mission, goals, and objectives been discussed by the steering committee?

¬ Have other program development committees discussed the mission, goals, and objectives?

¬ What process is used to validate the mission, goals, and objectives with staff or partners?

¬ What is the measurement process or reporting process for goal completion?

¬ Is the staff growth and development plan in support of the mission, goals, and objectives?

Political Questions

¬ Does the steering committee or program committee have any say in the direction of the program?

¬ What is the major drive of the program? Is this drive consistent with the mission, goals, and objectives?

¬ Are the mission, goals, and objectives consistent with those of health partners

(e.g., medical office, employee assistance program, and safety and health department)?

¬ Are the mission, goals, and objectives written in the same language as the overall company key initiatives?

¬ Do stakeholders feel that the program mission, goals, and objectives are aligned correctly?

¬ Are there any key company initiatives that the program has not taken advantage of?

Cultural Questions

¬ How do the employees feel about the company's value of health?

¬ What terms were used in the data collection process for individuals to define health?

¬ Are the program goals shared with all employees?

¬ Are the program results shared with all employees?

¬ Can employees state the mission and goals of the program?

¬ Do employees feel that the program has been successful at meeting its goals?

Program Structure and Strategy

Technical Questions

¬ Is a committee structure used to provide the program ownership and guidance?

¬ Are agendas prepared for committee meetings and meeting minutes?

¬ Are committee members given job descriptions?

¬ Is there a schematic of the program structure or model?

¬ What health or business models and theories is the program strategy built on?

¬ Are the components of the program strategy consistent to ensure long-term growth?

¬ Does the program staff have a growth and development strategy?

Political Questions

¬ Is the committee structure well organized to build support?

¬ What does the survey tell us about senior and middle management support?

¬ Does the company have a program participation policy?

¬ How motivated are committee members?

¬ Is the strategic process shared among partners?

¬ Are the program strategies consistent with the company's strategies?

Cultural Questions

¬ What did the focus groups tell us about the structure and strategy of the program?

¬ Do participants or employees understand the structure and strategy of the program?

¬ What do different types of employees (i.e., new, old, participants, and nonparticipants) have to say about the program orientation?

Program Planning
Technical Questions

¬ What committees are active in the planning function?

¬ Are plans well documented in the committee minutes?

¬ What data have been utilized for planning purposes (e.g., health-risk appraisals, health and interest surveys, management surveys, and culture and climate surveys)?

¬ How much planning is done with partners?

¬ What planning model is used to ensure consistency among staff members and programs?

¬ At what point in the program development process is the planning process initiated?

Political Questions

¬ How strong is the planning function with other partners?

¬ How old is the planning process or model, and where was it derived?

¬ Is planning done with the natural strategic partners?

¬ What is the follow-up to the planning process?

¬ Do staff members serve on other planning teams within the organization?

Cultural Questions

¬ What data sets help guide the planning process?

¬ How are these data put to use in the process?

¬ Once plans have been developed, how are they put into action?

¬ Are there inconsistencies in staff planning processes?

Program Marketing and Communication
Technical Questions

¬ What marketing and communication tools are utilized?

¬ Have participants and employees ever been asked to rank order the communication vehicles for best use?

¬ What do the participants say about the marketing and communication tools being used?

¬ Are the distribution systems working?

Political Questions

¬ What are the communication pathways being utilized to reach management?

¬ Are there processes in place that enable the program to be marketed to new employees or new departments?

¬ Are the program mission and goals being communicated?

Cultural Questions

¬ Are employees involved in helping produce the marketing or communication pieces?

¬ What is the perception of the quality of the marketing and communication effort by management and employees?

¬ Are there certain groups of employees that are not reached because of specific communication barriers (e.g., language, access, or material cost)?

Program Incentive Systems
Technical Questions

¬ Are the incentive programs tailored or designed for all program participants?

¬ How effective are these strategies?

¬ How are new employees or departments provided information on these systems?

¬ Have employees been asked to rate incentive programs?

¬ Are any incentives applied to team functions?

Political Questions

¬ Are program incentives tied into any of the company incentive programs?

¬ Are any incentive programs tied into partner incentive programs?

¬ Do managers understand the value of incentives?

¬ Have staff utilized different levels of incentives effectively?

Cultural Questions

¬ Have employees been used to help design the incentive systems?

¬ Have employees ever been asked what they would like as an incentive system?

¬ What rating do employees give the current incentive system?

¬ How important are incentives or the use of incentives to employees?

Program Delivery and Intervention
Technical Questions

¬ Is there a program delivery model?

¬ Is the program calendar broken down by program delivery model components?

¬ What is the driving force behind the program? Is it monthly themes or data?

¬ What level of programs is being delivered (e.g., awareness, screening and assessment, behavior change, or environment and support)?

¬ Is the program strategy designed to intervene at individual, departmental, and organizational levels?

¬ Are programs being well coordinated with partners?

¬ How well are the program materials organized?

¬ Is the assessment process driving the programs?

¬ At what stage is the self-care program development effort?

¬ At what stage is the high-risk management program development effort?

¬ What is the follow-up process after program delivery?

Political Questions

¬ Is the effort to coordinate programs with partners consistent?

¬ Are programs designed with specific knowledge and skill level advancement in place?

¬ What input do direct line managers and supervisors have on the program process?

¬ What input do partners have on the program development process?

Cultural Questions

¬ What did the focus groups or survey tell you about which programs the employees really liked? Which programs did managers really like?

¬ Why did managers like these programs?

¬ Are employees aware of the different program efforts?

¬ Are they aware of program results?

¬ What primary targets are these programs reaching? Why?

¬ What has been done in remote locations?

Program Evaluation and Reporting
Technical Questions

¬ What are the major evaluation tools utilized?

¬ How computerized are the program records?

¬ Are the teams' meeting minutes maintained in a file system?

¬ How often are reports required, requested, and provided?

¬ What is used to communicate to management on a regular basis the results of the program?

¬ Are surveys used after classes to test knowledge and skill advancement?

¬ Are surveys used to test motivation and confidence levels?

¬ Is an annual satisfaction survey utilized?

Political Questions

¬ Are partnerships and alliances made with stakeholders concerning the use and sharing of data?

¬ What ownership and turf issues have gotten in the way of data sharing?

¬ Are management's needs for program results being dealt with effectively?

¬ How are these needs being approached?

Cultural Questions

¬ In the focus group or survey, does it appear that employees understand some of the program's successes?

¬ Do employees understand the need for individual, group, and organizational success measures?

¬ What types of self-evaluation instruments are being provided to employees?

¬ Are too many goals being measured?

Data Analysis

Once the data collection step has been completed, data analysis is started. During analysis, appropriate descriptive and statistical techniques should be utilized to help prepare the data so that a reengineering plan can be developed from the analysis. Therefore, the primary focus of the data analysis will be providing a variety of views of the data that will help staff and stakeholders understand the findings.

The final report should utilize charts, data tables, and figures that are consistent with the types of data reporting done in the field of worksite health promotion. More important, the data reporting techniques should be consistent with those methods used within the company and understood by the stakeholders who will be reading the report. At Marriott and Johns Hopkins the team focused on preparing a PowerPoint™ presentation that had been requested by senior management. Before the report is prepared, staff and project team members should discuss the types of data reporting techniques that will be utilized and plan their best use within the report.

Project Team Report

The project team report should be organized so that it meets the major goals and objectives that were agreed on with the process owner team. The report will link recommendations to the major findings and provide a sense of the urgency and priority for each recommendation. An example of the communication segment of a final report is found in appendix 15.

Presentation

The project team report not only should be provided in writing but also should be presented in a joint meeting of the project and process owner teams. The presentation should be well prepared and practiced to ensure it will move the teams to the next step of reengineering planning.

In preparing the presentation, it is important to divide the information into

¬ what the audience needs to know;

¬ what the audience wants to know;

¬ the possible benefits if the information is presented successfully; and

¬ what questions the audience might have.

This format will help the team present content that is focused on the facts, benefits, and ideas that will support the recommendations. The group should rehearse the presentation and assemble a small but friendly audience for feedback. The presenters should not read their parts but use key words to help them remember the key points they will make. Define all key terms that will be utilized, and test these definitions with a friendly audience. Try to either video- or audiotape the rehearsal, and then listen for proper pace, volume, and pauses.

Many presentations fail because the rehearsal did not include practice with visual aids and equipment. After the rehearsal, affirm the presentation strengths and provide suggestions for improving weak areas. Practice truly makes perfect in group presentations (Anderson 1993).

STEP 3: REENGINEERING PLANNING

Reengineering planning occurs after the project team has turned in its final report and made its recommendations in a presentation to the process owner team. After these steps have been accomplished, have several meetings where the process owner team has opportunities to discuss the report results. When the process owner team is ready, hold another joint meeting and initiate the reengineering plan.

This step might appear like an unnecessary step, and many programs will skip this step and quickly agree to follow all the recommendations of the project team. Unfortunately, by skipping this step, the process owner team has a much smaller opportunity to gain ownership and commitment for the project. The major reason for their involvement is that they are the true owners of the processes that will be changed, and their participation is critical in planning the task necessary to accomplish the recommendations. It was this involvement at PSE&G that propelled the plan forward.

Project Scope

One of the first questions that must be answered in the joint reengineering planning meetings is the scope of the project. Two considerations must always be used to test the realistic nature of project scope.

¬ Can the project be completed on time or within the window of opportunity?

¬ Can the project be completed with the available resources (i.e., budget, people, supplies, and equipment)?

If a project is allowed to remain too broad, it could become so complex that it is too hard to manage and fails because of lack of support from stakeholders and management. Some groups simplify the scope of projects. These projects can spin off additional subprojects that can cause delays and increase the need for planning. Find a project scope that fits the program, its staff, and current group of stakeholders. Projects that are too ambitious can force regular programs to stop or have a negative effect on program quality. Teams that only take on small projects appear to management as non–risk takers or as teams that are not highly creative or innovative. Finding the right size change project for a team is part art and part science. Only experience can help teams develop the skills, knowledge, and intuition to determine the proper scope of a project.

Breaking Down a Project Into Tasks

Once the scope of the project has been determined, the project must be organized into work tasks. Breaking down work into tasks forces a team to see how things fit together in a project, how they overlap, and how one task might interfere with another. Tasking projects modularizes project elements into manageable segments, which allows tracking mechanisms to be set up that will help control and evaluate progress. It is only through the task process that the necessary skills and number of individuals requiring these skills can be determined. The most important role that tasking provides is that it ensures that all the work sequences are identified and understood (Baker and Baker 1998).

Network Diagram

Project teams must find the tools to help them manage projects effectively. One tool is a project network diagram that forces the project team to draw a road map of the project (see figure 17.02 for an example). This road map will include the starting and completion dates and names of the responsible team members completing each task. A properly sequenced network diagram will do the following:

¬ Show the sequence of tasks to be completed for the whole project.

¬ Identify the milestones that will be used to monitor accomplishments and progress.

¬ Show the interrelationships of tasks.

¬ Provide a vehicle for the scheduling of completion of tasks.

STEP 4: PROJECT IMPLEMENTATION

Several factors are very important to ensuring a successful project completion. The first step is to organize an implementation team comprising a mix of project and process owner team members and individuals who were not part of the original planning process. The size of the implementation team will depend on the scope of the project and time frame for its accomplishment.

Be a Real Project Leader

Real project leaders understand the difference between managing a project and being the project leader. Bennis and Nanus (1985) provided a clear difference between leaders and managers when they suggested that managers are people who do things right and leaders are people who do the right thing. A project manager is an individual who has responsibility and makes things happen, whereas a project leader is an individual who influences and guides the direction of opinion and the course

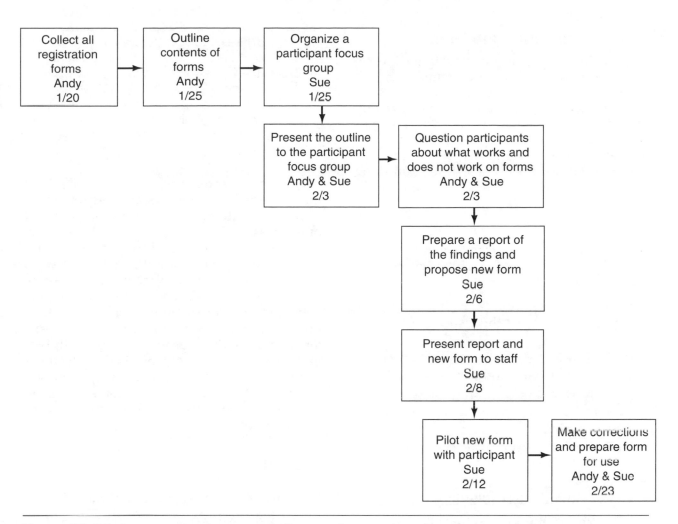

Figure 17.02 An example of a network diagram for a registration change process.

of action inside and outside of his or her team.

Successful project leaders increase their potential value and the project's worth by integrating these two roles. The synergistic relationship between leadership and management provides a balance in a project that increases the opportunity for project success. Gardner (1990) suggests that integrated leaders will

¬ act as visionaries and futurists who always consider the effect of their decisions in both the short and long term;

¬ look toward the larger organization in understanding how their departments' actions fit into the larger picture and not become narrowly focused;

¬ influence others beyond the organization's bureaucratic boundaries;

¬ emphasize vision, values, and motivation;

¬ deal with the many different expectations and conflicts that arise from their clients; and

¬ think in terms of change and renewal to help the organization keep pace in an ever-changing world.

Successful project managers create and communicate a project vision that provides a plan strongly aligned with the mission and goals of the organization and the wants and needs of employees. The plan complements both management and customer service philosophy to ensure the project fits the corporate culture. Strong leaders not only provide a vision for their team members but also help transform team members into visionaries. Visionaries are individuals who are willing to take risks and understand the necessity and importance of building partnerships and alliances that strengthen the values of support and community.

Execute the Plan

During the implementation stage, the reengineering plan must be executed in its entirety. The network diagrams that have been prepared will help guide the implementation process and ensure that high-quality communication continues among the different implementation teams. The project leader must be ready to put out fires that will happen along the way with tested conflict resolution techniques (Tagliere 1992).

Conflict Resolution Techniques

¬ Agree that logical disagreements will exist but that everyone wants a win-win agreement.

¬ Identify the issues.

¬ Agree to deal with the issues one at a time.

¬ Allow the first person to tell his or her views without interruption.

¬ After the first person finishes, allow feedback to be provided to ensure proper understanding.

¬ Have the first person correct any misunderstandings.

¬ Have the second person tell his or her views without interruption.

¬ After the second person finishes, allow feedback to be provided to ensure proper understanding.

¬ Have the second person correct any misunderstandings.

¬ The team brainstorms ways to settle the issue, recording the ideas on a flip chart.

¬ The team uses decision-making aids to help them reach a decision if necessary.

¬ The decision is recorded.

During project execution, the tracking and monitoring of the plan is very important. As different project milestones are reached, a process must be in place to monitor for deviations from the plan. When deviations take place, corrective actions must be taken to ensure that the plan stays on track and the project steps stay intact. Good project leaders can adapt resources, schedules, and project steps as necessary to ensure that the project continues to move forward without major changes occurring to the project outcomes.

In some projects, a team will be forced to return to the planning stage because the scope of the project has been changed so drastically. When this situation happens, take a close look at the project goals and objectives with the involvement of both the project and process owner teams.

When the project has been completed, a meeting will be held with stakeholders to provide an update on the project's process and outcomes. A written report should also be prepared after the project closure meeting with stakeholders that provides the details on what was learned from the project experience. Once this report has been completed, the project team can be shut down or disbanded. Many programs have project team members that serve loyally during the year to help the health promotion staff complete projects. Rotate these positions so that employees do not get burned out or find that their participation in program development projects is affecting their work productivity.

SUMMARY

Reengineering projects can breathe new life into a mature program and provide young programs a means to continue growing past start-up. Ten golden rules for reengineering project leadership have been adapted from Sunny and Kim Baker (1998), and they are as follows:

¬ Build the best teams you can.

¬ Define project outcomes early.

¬ Develop a comprehensive plan that you can monitor and update.

¬ Make sure the task schedule is realistic and has appropriate milestones.

¬ Define a realistic project scope.

¬ Utilize processes and tools that help your team stay focused.

¬ Remember that people must feel they count; keep them informed.

¬ Work hard at gaining and maintaining management and stakeholder support.

¬ Always be willing to try new things.

¬ Be a leader not just a manager.

REFERENCES

Anderson, K. 1993. *The busy manager's guide to successful meetings*. Hawthorne, NJ: Career Press.

Baker, S., and K. Baker. 1998. *Project management*. New York: Alpha Books.

Bennis, W., and B. Nanus. 1985. *Leaders: The strategies for taking charge*. New York: Harper & Row.

Bray, D. 1994. *Diagnosis for organizational change: Methods and models*. New York: The Guilford Press.

Gardner, J. 1990. *On leadership*. New York: The Free Press.

Hornstein, H., and N. Tichy. 1973. *Organization diagnosis and improvement strategies*. New York: Behavioral Science Associates.

McKenzie, J., and J. Smeltzer. 1997. *Planning, Implementing, and Evaluating Health Promotion Programs: A Primer, 2nd edition*. Boston: Allyn & Bacon.

Ralphs, L. 1996. *Organizational development: A practitioner's tool kit*. Menlo Park, CA: Crisp.

Svendsen, A. 1998. *The stakeholder strategy: Profiting from collaborative business relationships*. San Francisco: Berrett-Koehler.

Tagliere, D. 1992. *How to meet, think, and work to consensus*. San Diego: Pfeiffer.

Tenner, A., and I. DeToro. 1997. *Process redesign: The implementation guide for managers*. Reading, MA: Addison-Wesley.

Part IV Summary

New health promotion programs must be initiated using models that include best practices and processes focused on delivering results. Just as many businesses have used reengineering to return to competitiveness and higher levels of productivity, worksite programs can use the process to refocus their efforts on their clients and on obtaining program results. Process focus, management of change and risk, and documented improvement are the key elements in a successful reengineering effort.

Create for your program a sense of purpose that is linked directly to the things your organization has to do to succeed. The three-step process for creating and documenting a business-relevant vision for your department includes assembling your vision team and advisors; completing situation analysis; and developing, testing, and documenting consensus vision.

The five steps in the benchmarking process include (1) determining where to start, (2) forming two benchmarking teams, (3) identifying benchmarking partners, (4) collecting and analyzing the data, and (5) taking action to reduce performance gaps. Benchmarking concentrates on achieving superior performance and suggests that best practices should be pursued regardless of whether they are inside or outside the health promotion industry. Benchmarking works best when you can translate fundamental processes into a key business process, which allows you to cast a wider net when you are looking at best practices.

A case study of the Heart Check program, a seven-step model, takes a systemwide approach to improving organizational support for employee heart health (or any health focus for that matter). The model moves through a progression of measuring the construct of organizational support and providing easily interpreted data for company decision makers, from developing organizational targets of excellence, to linking financially relevant outcomes with those targets, to measuring the construct on a regional scale, and finally to developing normative standards.

Reengineering projects can breathe new life into a mature program and provide young programs a means to continue growing past start-up. Approaches to a reengineering challenge can follow several routes. One approach, the Baun Health Promotion Reengineering Project model, borrows from both the organizational development and health literature to create a model that can be effectively applied in worksite programs.

Part V

The Twenty-First-Century Challenge

Part Objectives

Purpose

¬ To provide readers with viewpoints of other movements that are influencing health promotion

Application

¬ Opportunities for health promotion in the next decade are not without some potential threats. Understanding the potential barriers will reduce the risk of failure.

¬ New communication technologies and emerging social marketing models of health care, based on the consumer's increasing influence as a key driver in the demand for services, is changing the delivery of worksite health promotion.

¬ The question of the direction of alternative or complimentary medicine is no longer a choice between modern science and ancient wisdom but one of combining philosophies in a new, richer, and more rewarding approach to health as a state of well-being and not just the absence of disease.

¬ Worksite health planners intent on supporting employees' search for health in body, mind, and spirit can look to the employees' communities as the primary predictor of their source of energy or stress.

¬ Many of the basic unconscious assumptions on which we base our health promotion programs in the United States do not hold in other countries around the world because our assumptions do not reflect the cultural priorities of those countries.

Vision

¬ It is truly the golden age of worksite health promotion.

Chapter 18

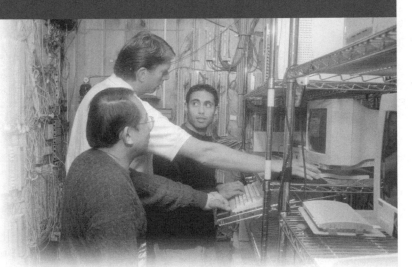

Introducing the Twenty-First-Century Challenge

In the new millennium, there will be many changes occurring in worksite health promotion. Following are some of the reasons.

¬ Competition for workers will force organizations to provide or expand value-added benefits such as health promotion.

¬ Quality of life will continue to become more important.

¬ Managed care will prove not to be the magic bullet.

¬ The convergence of advanced technologies and ever more sophisticated interventions will make health promotion more relevant and convenient.

¬ Growing emphasis on productivity will give health promoters a shorter-term metric than lowering health care costs.

¬ Baby boomers will aspire to better health.

¬ We will continue to know "what works."

These conditions will contribute to unprecedented opportunity for worksite health promoters in the future. Each opportunity, however, comes with a threat—a potential barrier or deterrent to success. The specific threats along with steps you can take to reduce the risk of failure are addressed.

COMPETITION FOR WORKERS

Salary and stock options are finite. Organizations wishing to attract and retain top talent in a tight labor market will need to offer services such as health promotion programs to address a top concern of all but the youngest workers (although rising health insurance costs are beginning to concern younger workers). Health promotion programs that are consistently delivered and in tune with what workers want will become part of the fabric of the organization—a reason to come to work and stay if all other things are equal.

Threat

Irrational Exuberance

The euphoric period of 1998 to early 2000, with accelerated economic growth and a dizzying bull stock market, produced a seemingly endless supply of money. For a brief time, it felt as if everyone would make enough money in the next decade to retire before age 50. Healthy people were even less concerned about future health than usual because money was flowing like water. Similar bursts of economic prosperity are possible in the next decade and will present the same distraction, relegating health to the back burner.

What to Do

Stop guessing at what your population wants. Think of them as consumers, and do your market research, just as you would if exploring the market for a new business. Ongoing needs assessment that focuses more on what people care about than what we *think* they should care about is the most effective way to capture their interest and engage them in behavior change.

177

Know that a brief period of irrational economic exuberance could be a distraction, but it will be short lived. Consistently providing services that people want will get your health promotion program through the unstable period as strong as or stronger than before.

IMPORTANCE OF QUALITY OF LIFE

The massive wave of baby boomers crossing the threshold to the second half of life will lead to introspection and exploration of life's meaning and purpose. As a large segment of the population grapples with the question "Is that all there is?" the realization will settle in that accumulating wealth and possessions isn't how they want to spend the next 40 to 50 years.

Threat

Disease Orientation

With some 125 million people (among a population of 276 million) in the United States with a chronic illness, there is legitimate fear that the nation is unprepared to deal with the economic danger this situation poses. As the fear grows, business and industry could develop a disease orientation to the exclusion of a prevention approach—undermining efforts to avoid chronic illness in the first place.

This disease-management emphasis ignores the almost universal belief that "it won't happen to me." By putting all or most of our eggs in the "fix it" basket, we virtually guarantee greater chronic illness that will need management—a much more expensive proposition than prevention.

What to Do

Disease management will help people and save dollars, so it should not be ignored. Be careful not to be lured into placing all bets on a disease orientation just because disease is an easy target. Instead, use the growing philosophy toward quality of life to attract healthy people *and* those with chronic illness. Your objective is not to fix what's wrong but to enhance their lives, add pleasure, inspire hope, strengthen relationships, and offer meaning and purpose.

Quality of life (including optimal physical, mental, and social health concerns) will become a top priority for many. Health promoters who position programs and services as improving quality of life—adding meaning and purpose as well as offering balance—will prosper from the population's philosophical shift.

MANAGED CARE

The initial cost savings of managed care have all but dissipated. More organizations will return to a traditional indemnity health insurance model or a hybrid approach that takes back much of the responsibility for population health and costs.

Just as it took most organizations a few years to shift wellness to their managed care providers (or drop the responsibility entirely), there will be some lag time before that accountability is reembraced. However, it will happen. When it does, we're not likely to see a return to large, internal corporate wellness staffs. Rather, we foresee small staffs who will purchase appropriate services from an outside vendor and manage outcomes.

Threat

Short-Term Focus

The "What have you done for me lately?" attitude of many managers and boards is not going away soon. So hanging your hat on the promise of cost savings from health promotion is the same trap it has always been. You will never be able to prove how much money you saved the organization last quarter (the time frame most managers care about). The best you can hope for is to present a convincing argument for *future* cost savings based on health behavior change results today.

What to Do

The cost-saving argument is the weakest leg to emphasize in a three-legged health promotion support stool. The others—risk reduction (as demonstrated by health behaviors) and valued benefit—are the real strengths of your program because you can show current success.

In quarterly and annual reports, your message should center on the health behaviors you have changed and employee support expressed for the benefit. Conveying this achievement with stories and personal anecdotes may be more compelling than numbers, so put them front and center in every management report.

Threat
Overreliance on Technology

Just because it is *possible* to do something on the Internet or with other technological advancements does not mean we should. Just because something is available does not mean consumers will want it. The landscape is littered with hundreds of dot-coms that have flamed out because no one wanted what they had to offer.

Health promoters need to be vigilant in guarding against the "gee whiz" factor, the "isn't that neat?" syndrome, and the "more is better" attitude that the newest technologies can engender. Quitting smoking, losing weight, or becoming more active are intensely personal decisions that may or may not be supported with technology.

What to Do

How you can appropriately use technology applications in your program:

¬ Go slowly. You do not have to be first to use every technology application, and you do not have to have it all.

¬ Look for technology applications that parallel success in the nonvirtual world. People still have to move, eat fruits and vegetables, avoid harmful substances, and get enough rest to be healthy. They cannot accomplish that through their cell phones or computer screens. When all is said and done, what does the technology inspire them to *do*?

¬ Introduce pilot programs for new services. There is a lot to be learned from real implementation on a small group before rolling out a new technology to your entire population. Take it for a test drive.

¬ Manage expectations. Technology cannot do the heavy lifting of health behavior change, and it will not solve all of your problems. So set realistic goals and build on success with each new application until you achieve the right mix of virtual and nonvirtual services.

ADVANCED TECHNOLOGIES

The tools available to health promoters today, combined with our growing understanding of how people learn and change, hold the promise for unprecedented breadth and depth of services. Interactive, real-time, personalized delivery of the type of health information people want has the potential to affect thousands of individuals at once—just as if they are sitting down with their doctor, dietitian, personal trainer, or health educator. This development can remove two big obstacles health educators have always faced: convenience and relevance.

EMPHASIS ON PRODUCTIVITY

Keeping people on the job and productive has immediate impact on the bottom line. This realization has gained greater play in the health promotion field because we have finally accepted the fact that we cannot affect health care costs significantly (or at all in a capitated system) over the short term.

Absenteeism, especially in tight labor markets, is a huge concern to managers. Demonstrating that your services either support keeping people on the job or prevent them from being off the job is a lot more compelling than saying your services will reduce health care costs over the next decade. The former affects them today; the latter probably never will.

Threat
Productivity Backlash

The least productive employee in your organization is not likely to admit that he or she is unproductive. People resent having others even imply they are not as productive as they could be. If health promoters suddenly add the productivity police badge next to the lifestyle police badge, there is a high probability you will turn off a lot more people than the couch potatoes who are not too fond of you already.

What to Do

Avoid or downplay the productivity tag, particularly when communicating with your clients. You want it as part of your official job description but probably not on your business cards or signature line. You want management fully aware of your contribution to keeping people on the job and as healthy and productive as possible, but if your clients perceive their contribution is being questioned, you run the risk of creating resentment.

BABY BOOMERS

Throughout the next decade, skilled older workers will not be forced into early retirement but will have the option to work full-time, part-time, or not at all. The massive population shift will present unprecedented opportunity for health promoters prepared to serve this market, both at the worksite and in communities.

Baby boomers will spend more money than any previous generation as they look forward to the second half of life. More than any generation before, boomers, not content to age as their parents and grandparents did, will aspire to a vibrant, energetic lifestyle. They will seek to maintain the vigor of youth for as long as they can.

WHAT WORKS

Thirty years of worksite health promotion practice has produced dozens of solid studies supporting the value of the discipline. There is enough data that health promoters in any setting should never feel a need to reinvent the wheel or be at a loss when asked to justify a program model, regardless of your program's stage of development (see table 18.01).

The advantage of knowing what works is that you can eliminate what does not work. For

---

Threat

Ignoring the Competition

Because boomers will be more affluent than previous generations, savvy marketers of all kinds of products will vie for the massive wealth this population holds. Health promoters who ignore the strength of those marketing messages could be left behind as boomers opt for the quick fix instead of the traditional incremental lifestyle change.

What to Do

Get out in front of the charlatans and hucksters. Be as aggressive with your message as they are with theirs but be careful not to cite endless studies on efficacy of the traditional incremental change. Instead, make your message personal with uplifting stories of real people. Focus on community connection, as well, to enhance life meaning and purpose.

---

example, a classic exercise in health promotion for more than 20 years has been to conduct organizationwide health-risk appraisals every 1 to 3 years. Implementation models vary widely, but often the paper appraisals have been distributed and collected by mail and then processed to produce individual and aggregate reports of risk. Finally, individual reports are mailed to participants or reviewed generically in a group setting.

Table 18.01

Pitfalls and How to Avoid Them

WHAT'S WRONG	WHAT TO DO
Ignorance. Most challenges we face have been tackled before, and we don't take the time or make the effort to find those solutions.	*Do the research.* Use others' experiences to help steer you in the right direction.
Lack of support. Because there hasn't been a strong enough foundation, sufficient resources aren't in place to do the right thing.	*Build your base first.* If you're lacking the money, staff, management support, or other resources to implement a program right, you probably shouldn't do it halfway. Poor results will only further hamper future support.
"Not invented here." This attitude is becoming less prevalent but it's still found, particularly in organizations with highly trained technical staff.	*Get over it.* In no other part of your business would you fail to use a competitive advantage—whether you discovered it or the competition did. Learn from others and build on their success.

An intended outcome of this approach was greater awareness of individual risk and high-risk behavior, ultimately resulting in behavior change and contributing to lower individual and group risk. It has not worked.

Consequently, individual follow-up methods for specific risks (and more recently, readiness to change) have evolved that *do* produce the desired behavior change. Today's health promoter can select tools and implement techniques with a proven record of success.

SUMMARY

All these forces (competition for workers, quality of life, managed care, advanced technology, emphasis on productivity, baby boomers, and knowing what works) combine to provide unprecedented opportunity for professional health promoters in the future. While not without threats to success, these conditions will prevail, barring some unforeseen major shift in the United States or international economy or some other change of global proportions. The decade will be seen as a time of accelerated advancements in health improvement, driven by a rising demand for our services and innovation from the bright, caring professionals who make up our industry. It truly is the golden age of health promotion.

Chapter 19

© Ken Graham/Bruce Coleman, Inc.

Using New Communication Technologies As a Bridge to Better Health

In his book *Player Piano*, Kurt Vonnegut envisioned a world split between the elite managers and those left behind. Worksite health promotion's future and the role of worksite health promotion managers may well face a similar split in fortunes if we are not prepared to rethink how we deliver interventions.

In the future, health promotion will be transformed in ways beyond our ability to totally predict. However it is perfectly clear that classes, printed educational materials, and fitness centers will not be enough if we expect health promotion jobs and health promotion programs to still be around. It is also obvious that just doing these current programs in a digital format will be no more successful. This chapter focuses on how new communication technologies and emerging social marketing and relationship models of health care, based on the consumer's increasing influence as a key driver in the demand for services, will change the nature of worksite health promotion and how we deliver it.

This shift is occurring for many reasons:

¬ Changes in population demographics and consumer expectations

¬ Revolutionary breakthroughs in medicine, although at a very high cost

¬ Employers reaching their limits as to how much they will spend on health care and increasingly diverting new costs back to employees

¬ Continuing development of new communication and information technologies

¬ A critical mass of communication technologies empowering consumers to take a more active role in making decisions about their care, moving them to the center of the health care process

Some may think the bloom is off of the digital rose. Although many dot-coms have met the reality of the marketplace, it would be a serious mistake to assume that the digital world and all of its forms of communication will not continue to grow into every aspect of our work and lives. Together, these trends are the ingredients for a revolution in care. When merged with theories of relationship marketing delivered via those very same "new media" technologies, these trends will be the engine driving the transformation.

New communication technologies provide cost-efficient methods for delivering behaviorally based health promotion and disease-management and care-management interventions to large numbers of people. Faster and cheaper is barely the story. Health promotion providers will need to customize interventions to make them meaningful to the individual, not simply provide a lot of static information, to generate long-term behavior change while creating the loyal relationships that are key to better interventions (see figure 19.01).

RELATIONSHIPS AS THE KEY TO WORKSITE HEALTH PROMOTION

In all sectors of business and industry, strategists are focusing on how to build more permanent relationships with their customers. Research shows that it costs far more to attract a new customer than to retain an existing one. Therefore, companies have become increasingly more focused on customer loyalty (Herzlinger 1997).

Perhaps nowhere is relationship marketing more relevant and urgent than in the fields of health care and health promotion. Yet, it is increasingly more common for patients to switch physicians, or even entire modalities of care (e.g., from allopathic to naturopathic), if they are not getting the type of support and communication they desire. Operators of health care systems in general do not have a clue that patients are customers too.

In her book, *Market-Driven Health Care,* Regina Herzlinger (1997) postulates that consumers will place a premium on having the ability to make choice and value trade-offs for their health care. However, she also points out that one of the biggest problems with the United States health care system is the lack of integration of services, particularly from the customer's perspective. While many of today's health promotion and wellness efforts are intended to be part of a relationship-building process, they do not recognize the needs of either the payor (employer), the provider, or the end-line consumer, creating a sense of alienation from the delivery systems of care and from health promotion as a part of the delivery system as well.

Alienation

How can we respond to this sense of alienation? We believe the answer lies in protocols that build affinity, continuity, and integration of services. We must place greater emphasis on communication that leads to greater consumer choice and involvement in their own health improvement and delivery in a personally satisfying way. Information must be presented in a context that is meaningful to the individual, a "microculture of meaning" (Newton and Sofian, 2002). American health care has created bureaucratic, financial, and language barriers to separate consumers from understanding and controlling their own health. The real power of the digital age may be its ability to reconnect people to those with whom they identify, while offering more options and supporting them through the care process, circumventing most institutional blockages that prevent each of us from taking care of each other and ourselves.

As worksite health promotion and health care delivery become more closely aligned, programs will benefit by adopting many of the

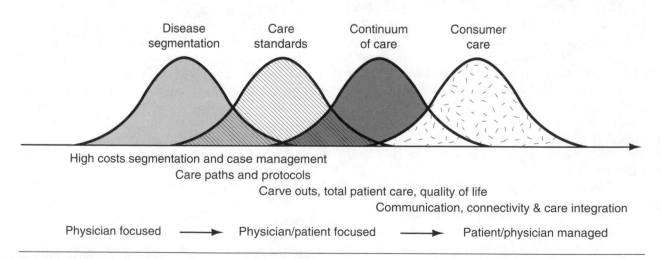

High costs segmentation and case management
Care paths and protocols
Carve outs, total patient care, quality of life
Communication, connectivity & care integration

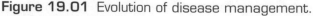

Physician focused ⟶ Physician/patient focused ⟶ Patient/physician managed

Figure 19.01 Evolution of disease management.

same communication technologies that are transforming the field of marketing. Advances in the development of sophisticated rule-based programming (also called "expert systems") now allow us to instantly and automatically find, tailor, and deliver very specific pieces of information to individual providers and patients—information that can be provided at work, at home, or at the doctor's office. Even more sophisticated levels of health care programming, heuristic systems that automatically change and grow in response to the data patterns that emerge through expanded use, will be available to health care providers.

In marketing, information technology is being used increasingly to determine potential buyers according to their "readiness to purchase" and other psychodemographic characteristics, to set the timing and intensity of their sales contacts. In the arena of health promotion, we can use psychodemographic profiles of participants to design protocols for particular segments of our populations well beyond the transtheoretical model. We can use communication channels, macro and micro message tailoring, and delivery formats that are most appropriate and meaningful for specific groups. For instance, a contact protocol may tell us when to send a letter rather than make a phone call or that a patient prefers e-mail to a group program. Taking it one step further, tailored messages can actually be constructed on the basis of whether a patient responds better to stories or simple fact sheets.

Increased consumer access to computers via the Internet and interactive voice response (IVR) telephone systems are hastening our ability to apply these marketing strategies. As of 2001, approximately 169 million Americans (60%) had Internet access either through their home or work (Nielsen/NetRatings 2001).

Growth in Internet use is expected to continue, driven in part by the convergence of computers, television, and telephonic and wireless devices, which will make the Internet more accessible to all. Companies such as AOL and AT&T Wireless have already teamed up to provide access to electronic mail, news, weather, MapQuest, Fandango, and MovieFone via cell phones. Numerous health care applications are not far behind (Barnes 2000). Also, as voice recognition becomes more prevalent, even typing skill will be removed as a barrier, creating even more demand.

Research also shows that increasing numbers of people are using the Internet for health-related purposes. Some 86% of people with online access searched for health information in 2000 (Harris Interactive 2000). Of this group, 47% searched for wellness and fitness information (PC Data Online 2000). Now this information can be tailored to match specific disease states and treatment options at a very personal level. Organizations such as Nexcura, on the basis of a detailed disease, personal history, and demographic profile, select synopses of the most current and pertinent research literature to assist in treatment decision making at the consumer and professional level.

With such widespread consumer access to systems that converge database information and communication technologies, we have the opportunity to increase the reach and richness of worksite health promotion programs as never before.

TECHNOLOGY ADOPTION— THE EASIEST CHANGE IS NONE AT ALL

While new communications technologies hold great promise, our success at effectively integrating them into health promotion will depend greatly on our ability to help consumers and providers adapt to change. Technology must be designed so that the perception of change for the consumer is limited, creating greater customer comfort. Amazon.com, the online bookseller, is a breakthrough example of this strategy.

Amazon.com captured a market leader position by providing a convenient new way for consumers to do something they have always done—buy books (and now other consumer products). On the basis of the idea that the most comfortable change is none (or as little as possible), Amazon eliminated the paper catalog but left the process of browsing intact. More important, Amazon is using each purchase (remember that a purchase is a behavior change) as a learning opportunity. Consumers see what other people similar to them are buying and even review the books for others to see. This creates a "microculture of meaning" where previously there was a group of strangers. Analyzing these patterns of data allows Amazon.com to increase its own ability to predict its customers' needs and provide products and services they may need but might not have even identified yet.

What lessons does this example provide for worksite health promotion? Employees who get one-to-one help with stress management, for example, expect to get more than advice. However, individual or even group interventions severely limit our ability to reach many people. They also do not offer us a systematic way to accumulate data to learn customer needs so that we can refine our interventions. Using technology to improve and leverage these highly personalized interactions, we can extend our reach and influence consumer behavior. Specifically, new technology must use data to dynamically impart knowledge, as opposed to mere information, to deliver personalized and interactive materials and services, not just static brochures or Web pages. Finally, new knowledge must motivate people toward health action and health-related transactions.

FOLLOWING THE MONEY

For communications technologies to become highly valued tools for worksite health promotion, employers will need to accrue both individual and population-wide benefits. Dr. Dee Edington has done landmark work in the area of health risk and cost, developing highly refined stratification models that use algorithms to identify potential high utilizers on the basis of lifestyle-related and medical utilization data (Edington and Tze-Ching Yen 1997). By linking intervention strategies to these data, we will be able to continuously fine-tune our interventions for maximum impact. For example, an employer, working with a health plan, could use health assessment data to flag future problems related to changing patterns in your diet, weight, use of medicine, physician visits, or lost work time and then select the most efficacious and cost-effective technological and behavioral applications to then intervene.

Consumers typically have access to computerized health-risk appraisals (HRAs) via the Internet or via the telephone using an IVR Touch-Tone pad. Soon voice recognition will eliminate the need for the Touch-Tone and the advent of Internet-enabled wireless appliances plus the perfection of Web-to-phone technology will reduce the need for full-fledged wired communications. All of these methods allow data to be trans-mitted directly and instantly into an organization's computer. Examples include WellMed's HQ (www.wellmed.com) Mayo Clinic (www.mayoclinic.com) and Inteli-Health (www.intelihealth.com). With the deployment of services such as Iridium, satellite transmissions will be available for the same purpose via personal digital assistants (PDAs) and wireless application protocol (WAP) phones.

For example, an employee completes an HRA in his or her workplace or doctor's office using a voice recognition instrument or hand-held device like those used by United Parcel Service drivers to keep track of packages or wireless devices such as Research In Motion's Blackberry. Computers receive satellite transmissions of the data and report them to a large database where they are analyzed to predict risk. An intervention report is generated, which is instantly transmitted back to all appropriate parties, tailored to their level of knowledge and learning styles, and allowing both health promotion and medical personnel to have the same critical data they need to deliver congruent support and intervention. Later, they will initiate reminders about health screenings and future appointments that can come via telephone, fax, PDA, or computer. Systems can even be programmed to send e-mail and voice mail to the participant or provider to encourage compliance as well as match individuals to others like themselves who are prepared to provide support and advice. For employees with complicated drug and diet regimens, pagers can be provided to the participant so that messages, directions, and reminders can be sent every day, throughout the day, wherever they are.

INFORMATION TO CONTEXTUAL KNOWLEDGE

As consumers become more knowledgeable about their health, worksite health promotion programs using technology will focus more on the quality of delivery rather than just on content, expanding the reach and richness of information they deliver.

TELEPHONE CALL CENTERS

Currently, most telephone-based intervention programs are quite similar to traditional classroom-based behavior change programs. Programs of the future, however, will become increasingly more powerful through the use of assessments to determine a wide range of psychodemographic characteristics. Assessments can be used to identify specific learning and behavior styles, as well as hobbies and effective metaphors for learning or to find others with whom to create an micrioculture of meaning support community. Participants might even take pictures that portray their barriers to change, describe their practices, or their greatest sources of support. These pictures can be placed onto the Internet, making it possible for them to be accessed by their phone counselor or shared with other participants through an ongoing Web log (Blogging). The counselor or other members of the community in turn can use this visual story to help create a more intimate, effective intervention process. Powered by such data, telephonic and other remote technologies may demonstrate potent outcomes, even stronger than face-to-face interventions, while offering vastly more reach.

Just as telephone call centers can deliver rich, personalized interventions to large segments of a population, so too will various forms of tailored communication, now available in a variety of media including print, IVR phone systems, and the Internet. Tailored health communication is an enhancement made possible through advances in mail-merge functionality and proliferated through developments in database and printing technology. Tailoring takes population targeting and segmentation—by-products of health-risk appraisals—even further to create "segments of one." Interventions are designed to fit each individual's unique set of characteristics and needs.

Most studies of tailoring health promotion interventions have involved tailored print newsletters, but a few organizations are also developing interventions for other media, such as the Internet and telephonic IVR. Examples include WellMed, a company based in Portland, Oregon, that uses an online HRA to provide users with customized Web links, pointing them to personally relevant health information sites (WellMed 1998). HealthLift, an Internet smoking-cessation provider, used an assessment to push relevant, highly tailored health messages, stories, activities, and illustrations to users via e-mail, tying the quitters to their own personalized Web pages, which are updated daily with ongoing progress assessments and activities designed in response to new status information (HealthLift 2000). Although today, most of this tailoring is print and visual, we can expect an increasing amount of tailored audio and video content that is tied to an assessment of the experiences of people who have successfully made these changes.

IVR provides an especially promising near-term channel for tailored messaging because of the population's widespread access to Touch-Tone telephones. In addition to simply collecting information via an IVR-based HRA, such systems can be programmed to facilitate ongoing automated interactions. For example, systems can be set to contact employees regarding medication regimens, their own behavior change goals, or upcoming screening examinations. Health promotion and disease management providers also can use IVR to answer consumers' questions with a series of personalized prerecorded responses. Using tailoring software, providers can mix and match those responses, creating speeches personally designed for a specific need at a specific time. In addition, providers may point their patients to an audio library of longer prerecorded programs covering a range of health-related topics in a variety of innovative formats.

PLANNER, TRACKER, STORYTELLER MODEL

Tailored messaging's premise acknowledges that effectiveness is often more related to the context of how a message is delivered and received by the listener rather than to the mere content of the message. In other words, part of making health behavior change interventions more appealing is to better match patients to programs, looking not only at how they like to receive information but also at how they are most likely to be "moved" by information. The

HealthTalk Interactive Case Study

HealthTalk Interactive, a Seattle-based company, creates a variety of interactive telephone and Internet "talk shows" featuring experts and lay people discussing topics such as asthma, headaches, multiple sclerosis, prostate cancer, and kidney disease. Shows are produced in a familiar call-in radio talk show format, allowing people to share resources, information; and most important, personal, even intimate, stories of how they have lived with health problems or made changes in health behaviors. A bonus is that, if the content is recorded digitally, it can be put up on the Web, eliminating all phone charges (HealthTalk 1999).

authors of this chapter are principals of The NewSof Group, a Seattle-based consulting firm that is helping organizations use new technologies to develop more effective behavior change interventions. NewSof categorizes how people typically approach behavior change in three different ways: planning, tracking, and storytelling. This planner, tracker, storyteller model is built on the understanding that there is no shortage of information in most fields of health behavior change. There is, however, a lack of insight about how to motivate people to take action.

Planners change by looking forward, setting goals, making plans, and following those plans until they achieve their goals. Trackers change by keeping records of their behavior and looking back and analyzing patterns. They then adjust their behavior on the basis of what they learn from that retrospective reflection. Storytellers neither plan nor track. Instead, they find the inspiration and strength to change by relating to and identifying with the stories and processes of others. They are first attracted by the emotional appeal of a personal story and then follow up by gathering information and strategies to make change. In the non-technology world, storytellers are the basis for Alcoholics Anonymous and many other self-help systems.

We believe that classic behavior modification techniques, which include goal setting, tracking, and rewards for progress, can work well for the planners and trackers. Planners and

trackers also seem to be a minority of the population. Storytellers may benefit from new and different forms of intervention that allow participants to share their own stories and listen to the stories of others. The critical issue is matching the right story to the right people to place the pertinent information in a context that can be effectively absorbed and acted on by the user. Patients can be encouraged to share their experiences on Internet bulletin boards, in their own journals, or by taking photographs to create a picture story of their barriers to making change. Search engines can be designed to match new users with experiences that will resonate with them. Telephone counselors can urge storytellers to see movies, watch television programs, or listen to tapes with narratives related to themes of behavior change. High-quality entertainment can arouse emotions, causing people to see their behaviors in new ways, thus enabling them to harness the emotional power that music, video, and personally relevant storytelling have to inspire and transform.

Still, there are people, who although physically isolated, crave the support of a group. In what might seem like a Star Trek experience, small groups or even single individuals can come to rooms that have "video walls." These walls are video screens designed to project what looks like a continuation of the room. When all participants are in their rooms, they appear to be in one single room. This arrangement delivers real-time sharing and participation although participants can be thousands of miles apart.

Consumers must have the opportunity, whenever possible, to learn in their own preferred style and medium. Ideally, tailored interventions of the future will be offered in a variety of integrated modalities. That is the intent of the American Heart Association as it works with North Carolina–based Micromass, Inc., to deliver "Change of Heart," a tailored intervention aimed at making lifestyle changes to reduce the risk of heart disease (Bulger 1998). The American Heart Association sends participants a printed kit that is tailored by stage of change as well as a highly tailored print or Web-based quarterly newsletter. The program also includes phone calls and reminder postcards or e-mail messages based on participants' stage of change during their most recent telephone counseling session.

Many other organizations are also using new technology to create online and IVR-based support groups that promote dialogue among consumers with similar health interests. People who share the same chronic medical conditions or who face similar challenges at making difficult behavior change can now find one another through thousands of online bulletin boards and phone messaging systems devoted to various specific health topics. In a Cleveland State University study of drug-abusing pregnant women, participants were eight times more likely to use the phone-based system than attend face-to-face support group meetings (Alemi and Mosavel 1998). The group who participated in the IVR program also had lower outpatient utilization rates, without bad effects related to health status or drug use.

The reach of the support group concept can be extended even further through the use of "virtual support groups," a concept being explored by The NewSof Group and the American Cancer Society. In this case, participants can use a toll-free number 24 hours a day to access the Cancer Survivors' Network. This IVR and Internet-based program includes 44 topical discussions categorized by age, sex, cancer type, and status (long-term survivors, newly diagnosed or in-treatment cancer survivors, reoccurrence, and caregivers). Listeners hear real cancer survivors telling their stories and providing supportive advice. People with similar issues and needs can also be connected to one another, create a personal home page to share their story, and share in a public "expression gallery," a space that allows survivors to offer up poetry, stories, pictures, and music. The overriding mantra is that all information for cancer survivors will come from other cancer survivors who specifically want to learn and connect "with people just like me." Callers also can be connected to the American Cancer Society's National Cancer Information Center for further information and support.

These systems can be integrated with other services because they not only track usage but also create detailed records of which segments users found interesting. The data could be used to generate tailored print materials with the customization based on which segments each individual chose to hear. To create further support at very little cost, tailored letters could be sent to phone participants informing them of other participants who have similar problems

or interests and want to be part of a support group. Such groups could become computer or telephone-based chat groups or in-person support groups. Either in print or online, these follow-ups could lead participants to other health-related products and services through the emergence of online e-commerce providers such as Drugstore.com. All would be self-generating and regulated by the participants at a reasonable cost if done on the Internet.

In addition, interventions produced as CD-ROM or Internet-based video games also deserve notice—especially because of their appeal to the learning preferences of children and teenagers. Click Health, Inc., of Mountain View, California, developed a series of video games in Super Nintendo format to help teach children to better self-manage their health, particularly in disease states like asthma. This form of patient education is clearly focusing on the needs of the market segment (children) and the way this segment likes to receive information (computer games and television). As this more computer literate cohort grows up, a games approach may become promising for all age groups (Chase 1998).

KNOWLEDGE TO ACTION, FROM CLICK TO CONTACT

It is great to describe cutting-edge technology that can integrate worksite health promotion techniques into seamless delivery systems, but with so much change happening, how can we know if we are moving in the right direction? The answer is in thinking like consumers.

When consumers visit a Web site to review health information regarding an emergent health problem, some health care Web sites allow them to make an appointment with the chosen health promotion specialist, allied health professional, or physician or order a set of customized self-care materials during that same inquiry process. When communication technologies are able to satisfactorily meet the customer's full set of needs during each health-related transaction, we will know we are building systems that are on the right track.

To achieve this level of service, communication technology will need to link information to program and medical access and to other transactions (behavior change, e-commerce). Before users finish their interventions, they must be able to get everything they need to take the most appropriate action for themselves. For example, an individual who has been recently diagnosed with diabetes uses a PDA to search information sources to learn about diabetes and complete a customized HRA. The individual might want to view choices for local endocrinologists who are a part of the employer-provided health plan network and schedule an appointment while still online. The individual might also want to purchase books on diabetes and a glucose-monitoring device that is designed so that it constantly downloads blood data, via satellite, to the individual's health record. The individual might want to hear stories of how other people with diabetes have dealt with their situations and connect with them for practical advice and support. In addition, the individual may want to link to the worksite-based physician's assistant to initiate an education and intervention process right at work. The individual is a smoker and is also enrolled in an online cessation program. The online program can connect the individual to professional support and other individuals who have faced the same issues and can provide meaningful alternative intervention. Finally, because the employer wants to encourage employee participation in these programs, all of the individuals' copayments are automatically eliminated and a variety of premium differentials have been added to the individuals' insurance as an incentive to participation in diabetes-related care.

From a behavioral perspective, each of these steps is viewed as a behavior, or an outcome. From a marketing perspective, however, these actions are viewed as transactions. When technology facilitates a desired consumer behavior and a consumer transaction, we are creating a truly responsive care system.

As this new vision emerges, it becomes impossible to tell where health promotion stops and health care starts. To be successful or even survive, worksite health promotion programs must learn to apply emerging theories of relationship marketing and communication. To capitalize on this transformation, we must do the following:

1. Focus on the reach and richness of content. (Information alone is not an intervention that will generate significant change.)

2. Think of behavior as a transaction.

3. Create a microculture of meaning. (Transactions work when there is a "real" rela-

tionship among the parties and information is provided within the context of meaning for the participant.)

4. Facilitate transactions so that we "close the sale" with a health action or medical event using the most appropriate communication technology available.

5. Focus on what people do, not what they say.

6. Start with the person, not the risk or disease.

SUMMARY

Technology integrated with behavioral science will be at the forefront of interactions between consumers and any aspect of the health care delivery system, whether at work, at home, or in the doctor's office. Facilitating consumer-oriented transactions for the purpose of creating sustainable relationships related to medical self-care and health promotion is the next wave in our approach to more integrated and consumer-focused care.

REFERENCES

Alemi, F., and M. Mosavel. 1998. Telephone bulletin boards reduce clinic utilization. *Wellness & Prevention Sourcebook*. New York: Faulkner and Gray.

Barnes, C. 2000. AOL Inks Deals in Rush to Go Wireless. *CNET* Sept. 5.

Bulger, D. 1998. Personal communication.

Chase, M. 1998. Can video dinosaurs help children manage illnesses like asthma? *The Wall Street Journal* Oct. 5, p. B1.

Edington, D., and L. Tze-Ching Yen. 1997. The financial impact of changes in personal health practices. *Journal of Environmental Medicine* 39:1037-1046.

Harris Interactive. 2000. *Explosive growth of "cyberchondriacs" continues* [online]. Available: www.harrisinteractive.com/harris_poll/index.asp?PID=104.

HealthLift. 2000. Corporate Web site home page. Available: www.HealthLift.com.

HealthTalk. 1999. Corporate interactive Web site home page. Available: www.htinet.com.

Herzlinger, R. 1997. *Market-driven health care: Who wins, who loses in the transformation of*

America's largest service industry. New York: Addison-Wesley.

Nielsen/NetRatings. 2001. Available: http:?209.249.142.22/press_releases/PDF/pr_010228.pdf.

Newton, D., & Sofian, N. (2002). *Microculture of meaning.* Seattle, WA: The NewSof Group, Inc.

PC Data Online. 2000. Online Study. Available: www.Newsbytes.com.

WellMed. 1998. Corporate Web site home page. Available: www.WellMed.com.

Chapter 20

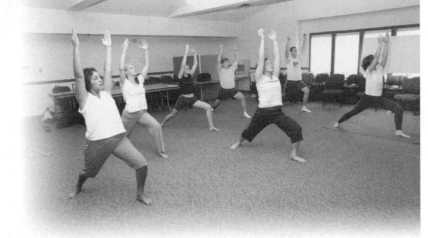

Using Integrative Medicine

If you want to attract the modern consumer, you must be able to offer options within your health promotion programs. Complementary and alternative health care services must be among those choices. For tens of millions of Americans, the question is no longer a choice of modern science or ancient wisdom but one of combining both philosophies in a newer, richer, and more rewarding approach to health as a state of well-being and not just the absence of disease.

HISTORY OF THE MOVEMENT

In the early 1980s, alternative medicine was considered "far out" of the range of normal patient care, and only those people willing to explore new territory were receptive to the possibilities of purchasing alternative therapies. Not until the National Institutes of Health established the Office of Alternative Medicine was any attention given to the developing interest in health care options beyond the traditional medical system. Even then, alternative medicine was conceptually "alternative" and questioned as "placebo or panacea?" By the mid-1990s, the descriptive term for these alternative therapies had become "complementary medicine." The terminology change helped to reposition therapies such as massage, relaxation, acupuncture, and homeopathy. Now, in the new millennium, the term "integrative medicine" is applied to the therapies and modalities that were once considered outside of traditional medicine. Interestingly, the traditional Chinese medicine model has always integrated those therapies considered outside the standard of medical care in America and other Western societies.

WHY CHANGES OCCURRED

There is a phenomenal purchasing volume of integrative medicine, and the cost is an out-of-pocket expense for consumers. Very few health plans offer integrative medicine services as a component of the health care insurance package. However, there are a growing number of health care insurance plans that are researching the feasibility of supplemental rider policies to the basic package.

Reasons for this change include the following:

¬ Public demand. Public imperative is driving the addition of integrative medicine choices. Most often, the consumer is seeking choices for back and neck problems, mood issues of anxiety or depression, burnout, or headaches.

¬ Dissatisfaction. Patients have expressed dissatisfaction with managed care plans and the minimal time physicians spend with the patient (12 minutes per visit).

¬ Mistrust. Patients have a growing mistrust of physicians and the health care system.

¬ Control and choices. Patients' desire to take control of their health, coupled with the health promotion programs that incorporate self-care and medical consumerism courses, is leading consumers to believe in their own ability to make wise choices in medical care.

¬ Experimentation. The baby boomers growing up during the 1960s and 1970s were categorically "experimental" and continue with that characteristic in seeking options in health care.

¬ Demographics and disposable income. The demographic changes to a population with many more people 55 years of age or older influence the interest in delaying the onset of chronic illnesses that have plagued many of their parents. Disposable income in this age group, as well as in the senior population, is substantial.

¬ Spending habits. The spending of the baby boomers is much greater than the spending of seniors who experienced the Great Depression.

WHERE THE CHANGES ARE HAPPENING

Hospitals have experienced an explosion of medically based wellness centers since the 1980s. Today, these wellness centers are incorporating integrative therapies, in which most participants do not require physician referral to receive the therapy. These centers offer "new age" exercise classes such as Pilates, yoga, and tai chi as well as therapies of massage and courses in relaxation techniques.

Resource centers at hospitals have increased prevalence since the 1990s and are tailored for gender-specific issues such as heart disease, high-risk pregnancy, and prostate and breast cancer. Resources such as clinical screenings and health education by means of video, audiotape, book, and computer are now available to the community resident. In both urban and rural communities, a person may access integrative therapy information at pharmacies, nutrition centers, grocery stores, and privately owned and operated new age clinics. Examples of privately owned and operated integrative medicine clinics are East/West Clinic in Denver, Colorado, and the Mind/Body Medical Institute of Harvard Medical School at Deaconess Hospital, which offers a variety of medical integrative interventions.

The greatest expansion of information regarding alternative, complementary, and integrative medical therapies is accessible on the Internet. Several information companies, publishing companies, health care systems, and individuals have established Web sites. These Web sites link to other Web sites for extensive information. The consumer is now seeking validation of the accuracy of the abundance of the information. Because the public wants and demands that science be applied to integrative medicine, they are looking to the health providers to sort the good from the bad, the safe from the unsafe, and the fact from the fiction. The abundance of information is an opportunity for the spread of misinformation.

Home-based health and medical information is developing as we enter the new century. In some states, technology enables the physician to monitor a patient's health status moment by moment. Information, readily accessible for the caregiver as well as the patient, is a major advancement, especially in critical life and death situations and in rural areas where it is difficult for the caregiver to be physically present.

The worksite of today is developing a different look. Telecommuters, flexible work hours, and decentralized worksites require additional efficiency and more effective means of communicating information. Corporate America is seeking improved profits, thus requiring health promotion programs to remain competitive with other corporate investment options. At the worksite, we now have four generations working. Each generation is differently positioned for health information. Each decade of a worker's life presents new health challenges to that employee and his or her family. The acceptance of the workforce becoming increasingly diverse in terms of gender, age, cultural, and language supports the idea for health promotion programs to accommodate the diversity. The worksite is evolving through mergers and acquisitions, reengineering, and restructuring for competitive advantage. Integrative therapies must be a component of all health promotion programs to meet future changes. Health promotion professionals have an opportunity to be catalysts and providers within the worksite environment.

INTEGRATIVE THERAPIES AND THE WORKSITE HEALTH PROMOTION MANAGER

Corporate America is competitive in the global economy. To remain well positioned, corporate leaders, health care providers, and health insurance companies must reconcile the demand–supply tug of war and achieve pricing strategies that are amenable to corporations, employees, retirees, and insurance companies. This feat is no easy task. To add integrative therapies as a third-party reimbursable item adds additional costs without measurable outcomes. Who is going to pay the premium? A transformation in the health care system needs to transcend into a delivery system that includes integrative medicine. Today, the greater issue is the significantly more demand than the supply can accommodate with efficacious, evidence-based research and practice standards applied to multiple therapies.

Some integrative therapies have attained the status of necessitating certain educational requirements, credentialing, malpractice insurance, and statutory oversight. Some medical schools in the United States currently offer courses devoted to the topic of integrative medicine. These courses are designed to provide physicians-in-training with sufficient knowledge and management skills to responsibly advise patients.

Policy changes have been presented to Congress and more are coming soon. In 1996, Washington became the first state to require reimbursement for treatment performed by any licensed or certified health care practitioner, including massage therapists, acupuncturists, and practitioners of some 30 other disciplines. Licensed, certified, or registered practitioners are the providers for integrative therapies and will continue to be the recognized providers. Policy, regulation, evidenced-based research, and credentialed practitioners will eliminate the charlatans selling snake oil.

FORECAST FOR INTEGRATIVE THERAPIES

The forecast for the development of integrative therapies is as follows:

List of Classifications for Alternative Medicine

This classification was developed by the National Institutes of Health Office of Alternative Medicine. The listing is partial.

Alternative Systems of Medical Practice

Acupuncture	Naturopathic medicine
Ayurveda	Traditional Oriental medicine
Homeopathic	

Bioelectromagnetic Applications

Diet, Nutrition, Lifestyle Changes

Changes in lifestyle and diet	Megavitamins
Macrobiotica	Nutritional supplements

Mind–Body Control

Biofeedback	Meditation
Dance therapy	Music therapy
Guided imagery	Relaxation techniques
Humor therapy	Support groups
Hypnotherapy	Yoga

Herbal Medicine

Echinacea	Ginkgo Biloba extract
Ginger Rhizome	

Manual Healing

Acupressure	Massage therapy
Alexander technique	Reflexology
Aromatherapy	Rolfing
Chiropractic medicine	Therapeutic touch
Feldenkrais method	

Pharmacological and Biological Treatments

Antioxidizing agents	Chelation therapy

¬ The consumer approaches illness as something that "happens to me" versus something that "happens within me." The physician's approach is to fix or cure the problem through the science of medicine, and the healing process will be as a partnership with application of all available resources.

¬ The physician will routinely prescribe integrative medicine therapies that are reimbursable through health plans.

¬ The physician will need to consider the liability of referring or not referring his or her patient for integrative therapies.

¬ The disease-management models will incorporate integrative therapies where acceptance is most likely to occur and then follow with integrative therapies that are preventive medicine and that promote health.

¬ New medical school curriculums will be developed with specific degrees awarded for integrative medicine and therapies, presenting an opportunity for health promotion managers to obtain dual degrees.

¬ The health promotion profession must consider standards, certification, and possibly licensure.

¬ Standards of care will be developed as double-blind studies prove the efficacy of different therapies.

¬ As with allopathic medicine, generalists or family doctors specializing in integrative medicine will appear as providers.

¬ The next generation, those born in the late 1990s and on, will be raised with integrative medicine woven into their care.

SUMMARY

The truth will only be known as time unfolds the direction, decisions, and desires of the consumer (patient), insurance, medical and health care providers, and the corporations who all have a vested interest in integrative medicine.

Chapter 21

© Bruce Coleman, Inc.

Expanding Workplace Health Promotion Globally

"The focus of this chapter is the 1.5 billion people living in developed countries because workplace health promotion can make a difference in the health of the people and the profitability of businesses in these countries. I spent one year in South Korea as a Senior Fulbright Scholar and have conducted health promotion–related work in about a dozen other countries, but by no means am I an expert on all countries in the world. Much of the following data were gathered through my own experience or provided by experts in the countries mentioned and cannot be substantiated in the published literature. It should therefore be considered with caution. The data are used only to illustrate the concepts. My goal in this chapter is not to communicate data but to stimulate a critical review of the issues by anyone interested in developing workplace health pro-motion programs internationally."

Michael P. O'Donnell

A quick read of the other chapters in this book makes it clear that we in the United States have developed an extensive science, technology, and discipline of workplace health pro-

motion. What may not be clear is that workplace health promotion has developed in the United States to a greater extent than in any other country in the world, and it is inevitable that other countries will look to the United States for assistance in developing their programs. The initial global expansion of workplace health promotion programs has already begun in global companies such as Coca Cola. This chapter reflects on how we must adapt our thinking to facilitate this expansion.

To develop workplace health promotion programs in other countries, we must do the same things we do when we develop programs in the United States—needs assessments. More specifically, we should get a sense of the causes of disease and death, lifestyle practices, cultural norms, demographics, workplace logistics, availability of health promotion resources, and economic factors related to medical care and productivity.

Approximately three quarters of the world's population live in undeveloped countries in Africa, South America, Southeast Asia, and some parts of Eastern Europe and the Middle East and in China and India. The majority of these people do not work in typical Western-style work settings. They often work on small farms, in day-labor jobs, or as independent merchants, or they just scrounge for food. Malnutrition, infectious diseases, lack of clean water supplies, absence of immunization or any other formal medical services, and

197

ongoing civil strife and sometimes war are the norm in these countries. Traditional workplace health promotion programs will reach only the upper classes in these countries. The health of people in these countries will be far better served through economic development, social stabilization, and basic public health interventions and community health promotion programs.

CAUSES OF ILLNESS AND DEATH

Table 21.01 shows the major causes of death in the United States, Korea, and Australia in 1999. These are three countries with significant differences in cultural norms, geography, population size and density, economics, and many other factors. There are some differences in the order of causes of death. For example, heart disease is the first and second leading cause of death in the United States and Australia, respectively, but it is the fourth leading cause of death in Korea. Accidents are the number three cause of death in Korea but are not in the top four in the United States or Australia. In Australia, water-related deaths (not shown in tables) are far more common than in the United States because most of the Australian population lives within 50 miles of the ocean. Despite these and other minor differences, the basic causes of death are strikingly similar in each of these countries. Lifestyle is a major contributing factor to most of the diseases in these countries and a major cause of death, as in most developed nations of the world.

> Health promotion can have a significant impact on the health of people in these countries. The relative importance of specific programs will vary by country.

LIFESTYLE RISK FACTORS AND CULTURAL NORMS

We need to measure lifestyle risk factors such as smoking, sedentary lifestyle, nutrition, obesity, and stress and cultural norms related to these behaviors. We will find significant variations in these factors across countries. For example, in Korea, the norm is that men smoke, and women do not smoke. Most smokers seem to be in the precontemplation stage and are thus not ready to quit smoking. Also, drinking is part of the culture. For example, at Yonsei University, the top-rated private university in Korea, the typical male faculty member will drink five or more drinks at a sitting on at least two nights of every week. A Korean man who declines to smoke or drink in a social situation will often be excluded by his friends. Tradi-

Table 21.01

Leading Causes of Death in the United States, Korea, and Australia

COUNTRY	CAUSES OF DEATH
United States (National Center for Health Statistics, 1999)	1. Heart disease 2. Cancer 3. Stroke 4. Respiratory diseases
Korea (WHO: World Health Statistics Annual, 1999)	1. Cancer 2. Stroke 3. Accidents and injury 4. Heart disease
Australia (Australian Bureau of Statistics, 2000)	1. Cancer 2. Heart disease 3. Stroke

tional quit-smoking courses or courses in responsible drinking will not work in Korea because most men are not ready to quit, and those who are successful in quitting will face social isolation from their friends and colleagues and probably suffer relapse. Historically, health per se has not been highly valued by Korean people. Political independence, working hard, being a good parent and productive member of society, and showing respect for elders and authority are far more important. Therefore, a quit-smoking program that stresses the importance of being a good (nonsmoking) role model for one's children, the economic cost of smoking to society, and the impact of smoking on productivity would be more effective than a program that stresses only health consequences.

In India, sedentary lifestyle is the norm, in part because of the Hindu religion and related culture. Within this culture, exercise is thought to be somewhat vain because building a strong physical body is not thought to contribute to developing one's soul. Furthermore, burning calories through exercise in a country suffering from extreme food shortages is sometimes perceived as similar to wasting water by taking long showers in a country suffering from droughts. Exercise programs in India would need to focus more on the impact of exercise on improving mental clarity, draw on traditional formats such as yoga, and downplay the "body beautiful" element.

DEMOGRAPHICS

The United States is one of the most culturally diverse countries in the world, with people from Hispanic, African, Asian, Middle Eastern, and European backgrounds. To be successful in reaching all of the employees in a large United States company, programs need to be adapted to be sensitive to each of these cultures, and learning difficulties related to language differences and illiteracy need to be considered. In contrast, Korea is a very homogeneous country with 95% of the population pure Korean. Furthermore, literacy rates are almost 100% among the population under age 55, and most Koreans are very good at sitting in a classroom and absorbing lots of material by rote. One program, sensitive to the Korean culture, will probably work with all members of society. In China, most of the population is ethnic Chi-

nese but because of the geographic dispersion, there are many subcultures and dialects, and programs would need to be tailored to each of these groups.

WORKPLACE LOGISTICS AND HEALTH PROMOTION RESOURCES

Most of our experience and success in workplace health promotion programs has been in large, centralized companies in the United States. We are often able to develop cost-effective programs by purchasing existing health promotion materials, hiring local venders to conduct screenings and teach courses, and spreading the cost of programs across many employees. We are also able to build fitness centers on existing land or in underutilized space within our buildings or purchase memberships at bulk discounts from local fitness centers.

In many countries around the world, it is not possible to purchase existing health promotion materials or hire local health promotion venders because they just do not exist. Furthermore, the structure of workplaces is different in every country. Many employers around the world have smaller or at least less centralized workforces. Land and building space costs are so high that it is often prohibitively expensive to build an on-site fitness center, and the space on which commercial fitness centers are built is so expensive that they can often be afforded only by the upper class.

ECONOMIC MOTIVATORS FOR BUSINESS

Employers in the United States have supported health promotion programs in part to enhance image, increase productivity, and reduce medical care costs, all of which can lead to improved profits. Many of these factors will not apply in other countries.

For example, in Korea, annual medical care costs are about $500 per year. The employer pays annual premiums of about $300 to a central insurance fund. Half of this amount is deducted from the employee's wages, and half is paid by the employer. When the employee uses medical care services, there is a copayment averaging 50% for outpatient services and 20%

for inpatient services. Therefore, the annual cost of medical care to the employer is around $150 compared with almost $4,000 in the United States. Not surprisingly, medical care cost containment is not a priority in Korea for most employers. In Australia, medical care costs around $1,600 a year and is funded through payroll deductions and general taxes. The employer bears none of the cost. The employee and the government may be concerned about medical care cost containment, but employers in Australia are not concerned.

Absenteeism is one of the few elements of productivity we have been able to study in relationship to health promotion. We have found that health promotion programs do reduce absenteeism in the United States where absenteeism is sometimes a problem. In Korea, absenteeism is so low that there is no Korean word to express it. Obviously, absenteeism reduction will not be a motivator in Korea. In contrast, absenteeism in Germany is a serious problem. Most employers allow 30 days of absence, and in the factories, absenteeism averages about 30 days a year. When General Motors built a plant in Germany in the 1990s, they decided not to tolerate these high levels of absenteeism and felt they could reduce them through policy change. They announced that any employee with more than 3 days of absence would not receive the winter bonus that is customary in Germany. The average absence rate of absenteeism in the next year was 3 days.

Absenteeism is a severe problem in The Netherlands. Most companies allow employees to be absent up to 2 years, and after that time, they may be able to go on disability. During this period, the government typically pays 80% of the salary, and the employer often pays the remaining 20%. The absenteeism problem is so extreme that an elaborate financing system, similar to the medical insurance system in the United States, has emerged to pay for absenteeism. Some scholars have devoted their entire career to studying and solving this problem. Absenteeism reduction will obviously be a big priority in The Netherlands and probably in Germany and some other European countries.

In Japan and Korea, the cultural norm is to work very hard for long hours. Very little effort is needed to stimulate people in these countries to have the desire to work hard. Health promotion programs, however, may be needed to give these employees the physical stamina to be able to work such long hours. In some of the Asian and European countries now shifting from a communist to capitalist structure, the concept of working hard for a full day is not part of the culture. Enhancing productivity in these countries would require a major cultural shift and, probably more important, a continuation of the ongoing restructuring of the economy. In some Latin American and European countries, there is often a higher priority on personal fulfillment and enjoyment than on working hard and making money. Employers could benefit from a stronger work ethic in such countries; however, the impact of health promotion programs on these cultural norms is questionable. Furthermore, many health scholars would argue that the lifestyle in these countries is really more conducive to health than the American work ethic.

The economic motivations to develop workplace health promotion programs will be different in each country and in fact may hardly exist in some countries. Each country must be studied to determine these motivations.

SUMMARY

Many of the basic unconscious assumptions on which we base our health promotion programs in the United States do not hold in other countries around the world because these assumptions do not reflect the cultural priorities of other countries. Therefore, the health promotion technology developed in the United States cannot be directly transferred to other countries in the world. However, the lessons we have learned in adult education methods, the health impact of lifestyle risk factors, risk-factor assessment, the science of behavior change, exercise, nutrition, organization development, facilities management, communication, planning, evaluation, and other areas of health promotion will provide an invaluable foundation on which culturally appropriate programs can be developed.

REFERENCES

ABS Statistics. 2000. Causes of Death. Retrieved February 10, 2003 from: http://www.abs.gov.au/ausstats.

National Center for Health Statistics. 1999. National Vital Statistics. Retrieved February 10, 2003, from http://www.cdc.gov/nchs/nvss.htm.

World Health Organization. 1999. World Health Statistics Annual 1997-1999. Retrieved February 10, 2003 from: http://www3.who.int/whosis/menu.cfm?path=whosis,whsa&language=english.

Chapter 22

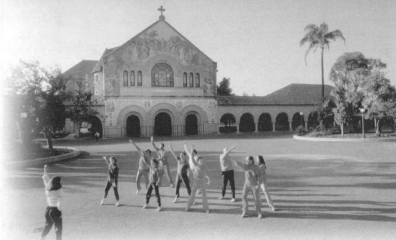

Providing a Broader Vision for Worksite Health

Improving employee health is fundamentally linked to the need to strengthen communities. Whereas our understanding of the relationship between behavior and illness is derived from health science, the worksite health promotion profession will achieve its greatest potential when it branches into the community. This chapter describes how corporate community service policies and programs complement employee health programs. Evidence-based reasons will be offered for why health promotion practitioners should provide leadership in community service.

COMMUNITY AS THE SOURCE OF HEALTH

Worksite health promotion professionals are familiar with concepts of integrated health and know that social, mental, and physical forces all interplay to create health. The role of corporations in improving social conditions has never been more imperative.

Worksite health planners intent on supporting employees' search for health in body, mind, and spirit can look to the employees' communities as the primary predictor of their source of energy or stress. When considering the resiliency of the workforce, preventing urban decay can be likened to preventing back injuries in the workplace. The one is accomplished through corporate service and philanthropy; the other through education and fitness pro-

grams. Both strategies are critical to the productivity and health of the future workforce. (Showstack, Lurie, and Leatherman 1996).

As a prime example, Honeywell, a large diversified manufacturing firm, offered comprehensive employee health programs for more than 10 years, including health screenings, disease-management programs, fitness and nutrition programs, and much more (Terry 1994). Honeywell also invested over 10 million dollars in housing redevelopment projects in the neighborhoods surrounding its headquarters. Working with city planners, Honeywell led an effort to demolish a one-block area of houses that accounted for 13% of the crime in the surrounding neighborhood. It has been replaced with Portland Place, 54 low-income housing units that have returned beauty and stability to the neighborhood. Honeywell leaders simply state that they hope to keep their business located in the city and believe that the company's future is tied to the community's future.

Whereas most worksite health programs focus on individual health, those with an appreciation for the powerful role of the community in shaping health must consider the corporation's social responsibility for health. Some corporations have entered health care reform debates laden with rhetoric about the need for greater individual responsibility for health. Some benefits packages were designed to penalize employees with high health risks.

ARISA-exempt, self-insured companies characterized such cost-shifting approaches as "incentives" that will motivate employees to improve their health (Terry 1994). In 1996, federal insurance laws changed to prohibit basing insurance premiums on individual risks. Still, lifestyle discrimination continues to be practiced by those health promotion programs claiming to support employees in managing chronic conditions, while at the same time targeting high-risk employees for penalties or rewards based on their individual health choices. Indeed, the nomenclature of "targeting high risk" certainly sounds more like taking aim rather than lending a hand.

Commonly accepted "demand-management" approaches are grounded in assumptions that individuals and their unhealthy choices are the reason health care expenditures have outpaced the rate of inflation (Breslow 1999). In reality, individual health habits are one of the weakest predictors of health services utilization (Kingston and Smith 1997). The clearest predictor of health status remains the social, economic, and environmental health of the community (Lantz 1998; Hart, Smith, and Blane 1998; Williams et al. 1995). Corporations with a broad perspective on employee health understand that health promotion and demand-management programs can improve the health status of many employees. Nevertheless, community and social factors such as affordable housing, job advancement opportunities, income, and education are the most telling predictors of poor health for many employees.

LOOKING FURTHER UPSTREAM IN WORKSITE EMPLOYEE HEALTH PROGRAMS

Competing for, and retaining, employees has become a critical skill for employers wanting to differentiate the quality of their products and services. No longer can worksite health managers be content with offering employee programs that every other company is also offering. In the past decade, employee health promotion has benefited from increasingly sophisticated lifestyle assessment and employee counseling. The era of clinical testing typical of the annual "physical exam" and the focus on executive health perks is long gone. Mature

corporate health programs will use sophisticated information technology to assess the prevention needs of their entire workforce, not just employees in need of special disease-management services.

Improving the health of the workforce has become not only a critical cost-containment imperative but also an expectation of employers managing self-insured risk pools. In the not too distant future, when company health benefits budgets are affected by larger segments of the population, using public health approaches along with tailored mass communications will be widely accepted by worksite health professionals.

Still, while these large population-based approaches are increasingly commonplace, many employee health programs remain fixated on the individual and his or her latest health problem. There is no end to the irony in the work of prevention specialists. The term "demand management" has come to represent contemporary intervention strategies targeted at individuals. The concept is limited as it relates to health improvement for large populations. If employee health improvement programs are to be cost-effective, increasing the employee's role in disease management will be imperative. Demand-management programs are reportedly achieving 7% to 17% lower rates of utilization associated with patient disease management instruction, self-care education, or nurse-based phone counseling interventions. Demand-management proponents argue that lowering demand for service holds more promise than containing the costs of service delivery (Fries et al. 1993). By implication, cost-containment strategies that focus on reducing the cost of employee services will never compensate for the presumed bottomless pit of employee demand for service. Such supply and demand logic, of course, positions employee health as a commodity to be traded rather than a value to be fostered. Choices become rule-based, and employee preferences are sought only to the extent that they can save the company money—not a strong philosophy for companies competing for valued colleagues.

Behavioral theories in health education assert that if people are educated about their personal susceptibility to health problems, they will be motivated to become more involved in self-management of their conditions. Companies that focus on individual patient behavior maintain that teaching employees to make safe, appropriate, and informed health care choices will yield a short-term cost benefit. This belief counters the argument that long-term economic benefit can result from programs designed to optimize personal health and well-being. When health promotion is positioned as a strategy for managing demand for health services, emphasis is placed on teaching consumers skills related to appropriate utilization. This orientation, however, comes at the risk of diverting scarce resources away from primary prevention education, which has been the mainstay of health promotion. This divergence in approaches indicates a need for role clarification in the health education discipline.

AN ADVOCACY MODEL OF CORPORATE HEALTH IMPROVEMENT

Most corporate health promotion programs focus on traditional risk factors such as smoking or obesity. Worksite health promotion professionals advance many health improvement initiatives by showing the relationship between risks and costs. This understanding of population health principles will also enable worksite health professionals to help companies understand the health improvement opportunities that reside in the community. Epidemiological data demonstrates, for example, that accounting for the cost of health habits inordinately shifts the burden of health care cost containment to the poorest and least educated (Sapolsky 1998; Gazmararian 1999). One study, for example, used data from the National Longitudinal Mortality Study, a survey base of more than a half million people, to demonstrate that race, employment, income, and education are the strongest predictors of early mortality (Hart, Smith, and Blane 1998). Looking at these community indicators rather than at health habits reveals that "targeting high risk" in the workplace should as often lead to low-paid single, ethnically diverse mothers as to heavy-set smokers. When considering cost-containment options, effective corporate interventions are as likely to be community based as worksite focused.

In the past, worksite programs were much more likely to examine what people do rather than how they feel. It is fair to say much more attention was given to the body than to the mind or spirit. According to one large epidemiological trial, women have three times higher mortality when they lack social connections such as family, friends, clubs, or church groups (Showstack, Lurie, and Leatherman 1996). Culture may also moderate depression. An analysis of the preterm birth rates of Latinas and Southeast Asian women showed that a strong sense of family and social support may be the most important buffer against the stresses of poverty (Guendelman 1995).

Addressing "nontraditional" risk factors such as isolation and depression will require action and collaboration at the community level. How the employee feels at work can only partly be explained by work climate. Issues no less provocative than life purpose, sources of meaning, and access to personal values are part of an employee's health agenda. When a company partners with its community, it is much closer to understanding these employee realities.

PARALLEL PATHS OF COMMUNITY AND CORPORATE HEALTH

At an educational session, this author introduced a role-playing game that simulated a company meeting held to advocate for a policy of allowing 40 hours of paid release time for community service. The "advocate" was armed with data concerning the health benefits of service to employees and the community. Other role-players in the educational game acted out the positions of typical company supporters and detractors of such policies. There were those playing corporate curmudgeons, ever wary of any activity that could detract from productivity or cost too much money. There were others who were mindful of the company image in the community, which could be both positively and negatively affected by community volunteers. Some roles in the game related to supporting the program for the wrong reasons, such as an excuse to get out of work. Others played roles of those genuinely interested in volunteering because it was the right thing to do for the company, its employees, and the community.

205

The parallels between trying to advance a typical health promotion agenda and the challenge of advocating for a volunteer program in the workplace were readily apparent to session participants. The role-players in the game readily agreed that the discussions that ensued from this activity were nearly identical to making the case for or against worksite health promotion. Just as there are those who believe employee health programs bolster morale, productivity, and reduce costs, there are others who think such programs encroach on valuable work time. Similarly, there are many who remain skeptical of the cost-effectiveness of prevention and the need for employers to accept responsibility for lifestyle-related problems. Philosophical positions concerning paternalism and the limits of the employee/employer relationships also emerged. This tension between private and corporate interests and individual versus social responsibility is familiar territory for health promotion professionals. Those who work as advocates of community service should find kindred spirits in workplace health promotion professionals.

Progressive companies will look for ways to address community needs in the same strategic manner that they plan health care benefits. Indeed, with employee health benefits representing one of the most significant marginal costs of doing business, employers may increasingly view community service as a means of protecting their investment in the company's greatest asset, its human capital. Still, other companies, despite compelling evidence that community health and social support issues are strongly linked to employee health, may view these issues as social service or medical issues outside of a company's sphere of influence. It may take public policy changes, such as forcing companies to share in the costs of care for the poor, to reconcile these contrasting philosophies. In reality, although the poorest employees in a workforce population may use health services more often than affluent members of the population, it may simply be a function of the fact that the poor have a greater incidence of chronic health problems (Showstack, Lurie, and Leatherman 1996). Some employers may see this circumstance as a need to "target" those with chronic conditions. It is more viable to conclude, however, that allocating additional resources to improv-

ing social conditions, such as housing or underemployment, would be more effective than investing in more health care (Barnett 1997).

BLENDING HEALTH AND SERVICE

As the previous sections illustrate, social isolation, depression, and lack of meaningful connections to a community are significant determinants of individual health problems. Disadvantaged groups in particular have some of the most significant preventable health problems that can be traced to socioeconomic inequities and the health of the community. Still, with health promotion professionals struggling to improve traditional risk factors, where is the incentive to take on community problems? When attracting participation in health programs is already difficult, why add another responsibility to the corporate health agenda? A remarkable synergy and mutuality exist between community service programs and health education in the workplace. In addition to the obvious community benefit from corporate service, volunteerism connects employees to the community and addresses the isolation and depression, the most costly of risk factors. Much more than stress management or other self-management programs, involving people in meaningful ways in the lives of others is powerful therapy.

Community service is also good for business. Marketing messages from for-profit organizations show consistent attempts to demonstrate their concern for the health of the community. Consumers are more likely to purchase products from organizations with a charitable mission. Similarly, nonprofits, abetted by tax-exemption statutes, are keenly sensitive to public trust mandates that they demonstrate charitable work and community benefit. The positive image of community service is reflected both inside and outside of a company. Volunteerism is a time-honored tradition in many companies throughout the country, and it is usually the employees rather than the employers who lead these efforts. Employees feel good about a company that allows them to serve others, especially if it is supported during company time.

Just as worksite health promotion needs both top-down and bottom-up support to be successful, community benefits programs need to be instigated by employees and supported by management. Moreover, similar to the most successful health screenings, such activities should be clearly voluntary for employees, but management can show that it values such activities by allowing activity to occur on company time. Although company release time is not necessary for successful volunteerism to occur, it is one of the most convincing ways to demonstrate that community service is a corporate value, a testament to the employer's interest in improving community health. Some might argue that paid time for volunteerism is an oxymoron. How can it be volunteer work if the employee is getting paid? The point is, corporate volunteerism is the way for the company to show its commitment to the community. Employees who wouldn't otherwise volunteer may begin, and those who desire doing more than the company supports will always be free to do so on their own time.

THE COMPANY AS COMMUNITY STEWARD

Collaboration and productive partnerships are watchwords of organizations that understand that population health improvement is a complex and prodigious task. Companies are clearly not alone in their interest in sustaining healthy communities. Health care organiza-

tions, nonprofits, public and private health agencies, and nongovernment organizations have population health improvement missions. No one organization can take the lead in determining priority community health concerns; rather, community health goals emerge from dialogue with community partners. Company leaders and their volunteer workforces can play critical roles in advancing community health agendas.

Developing employee leadership and organization skills is an additional benefit of corporate community service. Volunteers serve on committees, develop and coordinate special events, and assist with public relations and fundraising efforts. CCAs often sponsor educational events and volunteer gatherings that provide employees with an opportunity to share experiences and learn more about problems facing their community. The accomplishments of CCAs and their systematic documentation of activities afford employee health program planners the accountability they need to make volunteerism a supported and sustainable corporate activity.

With the goal to make volunteering possible for even the busiest individuals, the "City Cares" model of service is an ideal one for companies seeking to engage their employees in meaningful volunteer service in areas that they support, both geographically and philanthropically. Local CCA groups are organized to respond to the challenges groups and individuals have in finding time to contribute to the community when work and family commitments can be so demanding. The CCA Corporate Partners Program, in partnership with CCA affiliates, offers a wealth of resources, including knowledgeable staff sensitive to corporate cultures, a wide range of hands-on projects that address different community needs, and volunteer opportunities for large or small groups. CCAs also provide unique teambuilding and leadership opportunities, access to a network of affiliates across the country, and flexible scheduling and commitment levels that need not interfere with the workday. Working with an entity such as the CCA Corporate Partners Program will likely reduce the time-consuming and often costly efforts of forming a new corporate volunteer structure or developing new volunteer opportunities so that employees can participate in volunteer activities with ease and achieve maximum impact in the community.

City Cares

Abundant resources to support corporate volunteerism can be found in the numerous community agencies dedicated to enlisting citizens into community action. An organization called City Cares, based in Atlanta, Georgia, is a national service advocacy organization established to cultivate the growing network of local organizations known as "Cares" or "Hands On" groups (see www.citycares.com). These City Cares affiliates (CCAs) engage over 100,000 individuals in direct, hands-on service within their communities each year. These groups can work with companies to place employees in service projects, including house building and renovation for low-income and homeless individuals, tutoring and mentoring activities, providing assistance to seniors, working at soup kitchens and homeless shelters, addressing the needs of HIV-positive individuals, and coordinating outings for children.

City Cares Organizations

Hands On Atlanta, Atlanta, GA

Boston Cares, Boston, MA

Hands On Charlotte, Charlotte, NC

Greater DC Cares, Washington, DC

Volunteer Impact, Southfield, MI

Hands On Greenville, Greenville, SC

Kansas City Cares, Kansas City, MO

Hands On Nashville, Nashville, TN

New York Cares, New York, NY

Philadelphia Cares, Philadelphia, PA

Pittsburgh Cares, Pittsburgh, PA

San Diego Cares, San Diego, CA

Hands On San Francisco, San Francisco, CA

Community Impact, Palo Alto, CA

Seattle Works, Seattle, WA

SUMMARY

Employee health improvement strategies are vital components of a company health benefits program, but such efforts are "downstream" of the major causes of premature disease, disability, and death. Common risk factors such as smoking, poor diet, lack of exercise, and excess alcohol use explain nearly 40% of the major causes of death. Such risk factors have social, behavioral, and environmental antecedents. It is the community that is the keeper of these antecedents. It is in our neighborhoods and schools where healthful or deleterious life choices are cultivated. Progressive companies will be vigilant about their long-term plans and the needs of their employees long into the future but will also focus on today's unsolved problems. Socially conscious employers will see community problems as business opportunities and will learn that without concomitant attention to societal needs, their efforts to ameliorate individual health risks and costs will be ineffective.

A writing from the Sufi proclaims that "Today well lived makes every yesterday a dream of happiness and every tomorrow a vision of hope." Such is the promise of including community service in employees' health improvement programs. However, the monumental challenge of improving population health will not be met if the worksite health promotion agenda does not move at a more exponential pace. It will be the most judicious organizations that can balance the pressure of a competitive corporate culture with tenets of corporate social responsibility. John Lennon sang that the "love you take is equal to the love you make." Companies will benefit from the best communities have to offer when the companies offer the communities their best.

REFERENCES

Barnett, K. 1997. *The future of community benefit programming*. Berkeley, CA: The Public Health Institute.

Breslow, L. 1999. From disease prevention to health promotion. *Journal of the American Medical Association* 281:1030-1033.

Fries, J., C. Koop, J. Sokolov, C. Beadle, and D. Wright. 1993. Beyond health promotion: Reducing the need and demand for medical care. *Health Affairs* 17:70-85.

Gazmararian, J.A. 1999. Health literacy among Medicare enrollees in a managed care organization. *Journal of the American Medical Association* 281:545-551.

Guendelman, S. 1995. *Immigrants may hold clues to protecting health during pregnancy*. Wellness Lecture Series: The California Wellness Association. Woodland Hills, CA.

Hart, C.L., G.D. Smith, and D. Blane. 1998. Inequities in mortality by social class measured at three stages of the lifecourse. *American Journal of Public Health* 88:471-474.

Kingston, R.S., and J.P. Smith. 1997. Socioeconomic status and racial and ethnic differences in functional status associated with chronic diseases. *American Journal of Public Health* 87:805-810.

Lantz, P.M. 1998. Socioeconomic factors, health behaviors and mortality. Results from a nationally representative prospective study of U.S. adults. *Journal of the American Medical Association* 279:1703-1706.

Sapolsky, R. 1998. How the other half heals. *Discover*, April, 46-52.

Showstack, J., N. Lurie, and S. Leatherman. 1996. Health of the public: The private sector challenge. *Journal of the American Medical Association* 276:1071-1075.

Terry, P.E. 1994. A case for no-fault health insurance: From the "worried well" to the "guilty ill." *American Journal of Health Promotion* 8:165-167.

Williams, M.V., R.M. Parker, D.W. Baker, N.S. Parikh, K. Pitkin, W.C. Coats, and J.R. Nurss. 1995. Inadequate functional health literacy among patients at two public hospitals. *Journal of the American Medical Association* 274:1677-1682.

Part V Summary

The next 10 years will be the golden age of worksite health promotion because of issues related to competition for workers, quality of life, managed care, advanced technology, emphasis on productivity, baby boomers, and knowing what works.

New communication technologies and emerging social marketing and relationship models of health care will change the nature of worksite health promotion and how we deliver it. As worksite health promotion and health care delivery become more closely aligned, programs will benefit by adopting many of the same communication technologies that are transforming the field of marketing, such as tailoring health messages. Part of making behavior change interventions more appealing is to better match patients to programs, looking not only at how they like to receive information but also at how they are most likely to be "moved" by information.

If you want to attract the modern consumer, you must be able to offer integrative medicine options within your health promotion programs. In the future, disease-management models will incorporate integrative therapies where acceptance is most likely to occur.

Worksite health promotion has developed in the United States to a greater extent than in any other country in the world, and it is inevitable that other countries will look to the United States for assistance in developing their programs. The initial global expansion of workplace health promotion programs has already begun in many global companies.

The role of corporations in improving social conditions has never been more imperative. Risk factors have social, behavioral, and environmental antecedents, and it is the community that is the keeper of these antecedents. Progressive companies include community service in employee health improvement programs and look for ways to address community needs in the same strategic manner that they plan health care benefits.

Appendixes

Appendix 1

CHECKLIST FOR SELECTING
HEALTH PROMOTION VENDORS

Yes = **Yes, the vendor does/did this.**   NA = **Not applicable**

No = **No, the vendor does not/did not do this.**   NS = **Not sure**

1. INITIAL EXPERIENCE WITH VENDOR	YES	NO	NA/NS	COMMENTS
A. Did the vendor present a good professional image?				
B. Did the vendor do his/her homework on your company prior to the initial meeting?				
C. Is the vendor's philosophy of health promotion consistent with that of your company's philosophy?				
D. Can the vendor explain why his/her product is appropriate for your company?				
E. Did the vendor appear responsive to your company?				
F. Did the vendor explain how his/her product can meet the needs of your company?				
G. Was the vendor willing to listen to you or was he/she too busy trying to sell his/her product?				
H. Is the vendor willing to make a presentation to your company's management?				
I. Did the vendor demonstrate his/her organization's expertise with regard to the product?				
J. Did the vendor provide you with a reference list of other customers?				
K. Did the vendor leave written materials that summarize his/her product?				
2. PRODUCT QUALITY				
A. Did the vendor provide an overview of the product content?				
B. Can the vendor provide careful documentation of product effectiveness?				
C. Does the vendor have evaluative data to back up the product?				
D. Does the vendor have data to compare success rates of the product to those of his/her competitors?				

213

	YES	NO	NA/NS	COMMENTS

E. Can the vendor provide data that show the adequacy of his/her products with a population similar to yours?

F. Can the vendor provide several different products (health promotion activities) or does he/she just specialize in one area?

G. Did the vendor explain the types of interventions (e.g., behavior, aversive techniques) that are used with the product?

H. Will the vendor customize the product to meet the needs of your company?

I. Can the vendor offer a variety of interventions (e.g., different approaches to smoking cessation) from which you can choose to best meet the needs of your employees?

J. Can the vendor offer a product that can meet special needs of your employees (e.g., reading levels, various levels of health status)?

K. When appropriate, does the vendor provide written instructional materials to accompany the product?

L. If written informational materials are provided, are they written clearly and presented in an attractive way?

3. INDIVIDUALS WHO PROVIDE THE SERVICE

A. What type of education and training do the staff and instructors have?

B. Are the instructors certified by a professional or health organization?

C. Are the instructors required to update their training periodically?

D. Are the instructor-to-participant ratios reasonable?

4. PRODUCT DELIVERY AND SERVICE

A. Can the vendor put in writing the actual services that will be provided?

B. If a written presentation of services is made, does it spell out the responsibilities of both parties?

C. Is the vendor willing to market the product inside your company?

D. Does purchase of the product include an evaluation?

	YES	NO	NA/NS	COMMENTS

E. Can the vendor appropriately serve the size of your company's population?

F. Can the vendor provide the product at all sites desired?

G. Can the vendor provide the product at all times desired?

H. Are the lengths of the product sessions appropriate for your workday?

I. Does the vendor provide you with the name of one of their employees who can act as a troubleshooter?

J. Can the vendor also provide other products or services to other departments or units (e.g., the safety division, health policy) in your company?

K. Has the vendor been in business for at lease 5 years?

L. Is the vendor's company well managed and financially sound?

M. Does the vendor enjoy a good reputation in the community?

5. PRODUCT COST

A. Is the cost of the product competitive with the cost of similar products from other vendors?

B. Does the vendor provide written bids for the product?

C. Does the cost per unit go down when the number of participants increases?

D. Does the cost per unit go down if additional products are purchased from the same vendor?

E. Does the vendor offer corporate discounts?

6. GENERAL CONCERNS

A. Does the vendor carry adequate liability insurance?

B. Does the vendor put in writing a "statement of reasonable expectations" for the product?

C. Is the vendor willing to sign a contract?

D. If you buy the product of this vendor, will it improve the image of your company in the community?

E. If you buy the product of this vendor, will it improve the image of your company with employees?

Adapted, by permission, from J.H. Harris, J.R. McKenzie, and W.B. Zuti, 2002, "Anybody out there?" *Absolute Advantage* 2(2): 6-9.

Appendix 2

VALUABLE DATA IN EVALUATING HEALTH PROMOTION PROGRAMS

I. PERSONNEL DATA

A. Personal Information
1. Employee social security number
2. Employee name (last, first, middle)

B. Demographic Information
1. Employee gender
2. Employee status
3. Employee date of birth
4. Family status
5. Job classification
6. Employee race
7. Employee date of birth
8. Employment status
9. Marital status
10. Number of dependents
11. Employee education level

C. Election Information (Medical Insurance Selection)
1. Effective data
2. Premium cost
3. Medical option

II. MEDICAL INSURANCE CLAIMS DATA

A. Personal Information
1. Employee social security number
2. Claimant names
3. Employee name

B. Demographic Information
1. Employee status
2. Claimant date of birth
3. Claimant status
4. Employee gender

C. Claims Information
1. Cause of claim
2. Multiple service type
3. Service from date
4. Days paid
5. Service charge
6. Type of service
7. Diagnosis (ICD-9)
8. Service to date
9. Payee type
10. Amounts paid

III. HEALTH-RISK ASSESSMENT DATA

A. Personal Information
1. Name
2. Location code
3. Social security number
4. Department number

B. Demographic Characteristics
1. Gender
2. Age
3. Schooling completed
4. Expected annual household income
5. Race
6. Current marital status
7. Employee status

C. Physiological Measurements

1. Height
2. Blood pressure
3. HDL cholesterol
4. Weight
5. Total cholesterol

D. Psychological Perceptions

1. Self-described physical health
2. Job satisfaction
3. Personal loss
4. Life satisfaction
5. Social ties

E. Lifestyle Habits

1. Use of tobacco
2. Use of drugs or medication
3. Seat belt use
4. Sleep at night
5. Annual rectal examination
6. Breast examination frequency
7. Use of alcohol
8. Miles driven
9. Physical activity level
10. Violent argument
11. Pap smear frequency

F. Personal Health Histories

1. Diabetes
2. Rectal growth
3. Had a hysterectomy
4. Serious medical problems
5. Rectal bleeding
6. Chronic bronchitis or emphysema
7. Pap smear
8. Days missed work because of illness

G. Family Health History

1. Parental heart disease
2. Relative breast cancer
3. Relative diabetes
4. Relative other diseases

H. Wellness Program Participation Data

1. Participant identification
2. Program participation status for each program

I. Absenteeism Data

1. Employee sickness
2. Employee maternity
3. Family member sickness
4. Employee injury

J. Workers' Compensation

K. Employee Surveys

L. Employee Medical Surveillance Data

M. Other Relevant Data

Appendix 3

SELECTING AN ASSESSMENT TOOL

The following lists key questions to address in the selection of a health-risk appraisal. The source is the *Society of Prospective Medicine's Handbook of Health Assessment Tools.*

SERVICES NEEDED

In what formats is the instrument available?

How will questionnaire and results be handled?

What assistance is provided for promotion?

Is toll-free phone assistance available for participants?

Does the vendor provide orientation, counseling, or feedback sessions?

Does the vendor have additional educational capabilities for periodic follow-up?

SCIENCE BASE

What is the availability of the information about the science base?

Is the health-risk appraisal qualitative or quantitative?

Is the vendor using its own database? Where did it come from? How was it created?

Does the database reflect biases (i.e., socioeconomic, regional)?

How often is the database updated?

How are risks classified as high, moderate, or low?

Are morbidity and mortality data used?

What physiological data can be used?

USER FRIENDLINESS

Will participants find the tool easy to complete?

Which method will be easiest to obtain information (i.e., phone, paper and pencil, or computer)?

Are the instructions clear for completing and returning the questionnaire?

Is the reading level appropriate for the intended audience?

Is the questionnaire visually appealing to the participant?

Has the vendor produced the tool in other languages?

Can the vendor support customers' needs to be sensitive to specific cultures or subcultures?

How much time is required to complete the questionnaire?

What is the process used for distribution and collection of the questionnaires and results?

SCOPE

Is the breadth and variation of health topics covered appropriate for the intended audience?

Can the questions be customized to include client-specific questions?

Does the questionnaire contain educational value even if not returned for processing?

INDIVIDUAL RESULTS

How are results distributed?

Are the printed results appealing, and do they encourage participant use?

Does the report balance the use of text, numbers, statistics, and graphics to encourage use by participants?

Will participants be able to understand terminology and graphics?

Are recommendations provided? How are they presented? Are recommendations consistent?

What percentage of the results are customized to the participant?

If assessment is to be used over time, can the database compare for the individual changes over time?

AGGREGATE/GROUP DATA

Who owns the data once the health-risk appraisal has been completed?

Who are the data contact people for the organization?

In what formats will the aggregate data be made available?

How will the data interface with other health management data within the organization?

What aggregate tabulation and analysis can be done without customization?

Given confidentiality safeguards, can data actually be imported into databases of the client organization?

What is the vendor's capability to create customized group reports?

Are there provisions so subgroups can be analyzed?

What kind of training and support does the vendor provide in this area?

Is pooled data available for benchmarking?

Can the database compare changes in the population over time?

SYSTEMS CONSIDERATIONS

What kind of systems adaptations will the purchasing company need to make?

What are the staffing, hardware, and software considerations?

Does the vendor operate on a single or multiple platforms?

What are the operating systems and databases?

What are the vendors' plans for upgrading their systems?

What implications will this upgrade have on the purchaser?

How are data backed-up, stored, and retained for future comparison?

CUSTOMER SERVICE

How much time and energy is spent by the vendor to understand the purchasing organization's needs?

Who represents the vendor in these discussions?

What is the accessibility of staff with different expertise to provide ongoing customer support?

What are the expected turnaround times for individual reports, group reports, and customized reports?

How is confidentiality maintained?

What trademark and licensing issues exist in customization matters?

VENDOR–PURCHASER MATCH

Do the credentials of the vendor's staff match the needs of the purchasing organization?

What is the depth of knowledge by the vendor around instrument design and validation, program cost measurement, and outcomes?

Can the vendor meet the purchaser's need for scientific or business assistance in program design, implementation, or interpretation of aggregate data?

How strong are the vendor's information systems capabilities?

How does the vendor incorporate state-of-the-art communications techniques?

For what similar organizations has the vendor provided products and services?

From the Society of Prospective Medicine, 1999, *Handbook of Health Assessment Tools*; The Society of Prospective Medicine, 1999, *SPM Handbook of Health Assessment Tools*; The Society of Prospective Medicine, 1999, Institute for Health and Productivity Management.

Appendix 4

SOURCES FOR SCREENING STANDARDS/RECOMMENDATIONS

United States Preventive Services Task Force
Guide to Clinical Preventive Services, 2nd edition
Baltimore: Williams and Wilkins, 1996

American Cancer Society
Phone: 1-800-ACS-2345
Internet: www.cancer.org

National Cancer Institute
Department of Health and Human Services
National Institutes of Health
Phone: 1-800-4 CANCER
Internet: www.nci.nih.gov

National Cholesterol Education Program
National Heart, Lung, and Blood Institute Information Center
Phone: 301-592-8573
Fax: 301-592-8563
e-mail: NHLBIinfo@rover.nhlbi.nih.gov
Internet: www.nhlbi.nih.gov

The Sixth Report of the Joint National Committee on the Prevention, Detection, Evaluation, and Treatment of High Blood Pressure
Archives of Internal Medicine
Volume 157, November 24, 1997
pp. 2413-2446
Internet: archinte.ama-assn.org

YMCA
The Fitness Specialist Training Notebook
YMCA Program Store
Box 5077
Champaign, IL 61820
Phone: 1-800-747-0089

Cooper Institute for Aerobics Research
The Physical Fitness Specialist Training Manual
Fitstop Bookstore
Phone: 1-800-635-7050
Internet: www.cooperinst.org

Advanced Fitness Assessment and Exercise Prescription, 3rd edition
Vivian H. Heyward
Human Kinetics
Internet: www.HumanKinetics.com

Appendix 5

INTERVIEW GUIDELINES

Position: _____

Applicant's name: _____

Interviewer's title: _____ Date: _____

Other information: _____

PREPARATION CHECKLIST

☑ Review application materials for past jobs and experiences that are most relevant to the interview. Record the names of these previous jobs and experiences in the Key Background Review section of this Interview Guide. Start with the oldest job or experience and work toward the present.

☑ Review definitions of target dimensions in the Planned Question section of this Interview Guide.

☑ Make an estimate of the time that will be available to cover each dimension.

OUTLINE FOR OPENING AN INTERVIEW

Greet the applicant, giving name and position.

Explain the purposes of the interview:

1. To acquaint the interviewer and the applicant.

2. To help the organization make a fair decision.

3. To help the applicant understand the organization and the position.

DESCRIBE THE INTERVIEW PLAN

1. Brief the reviewer of past jobs and experiences.

2. Ask questions to get specific information about those jobs and experiences.

3. Give information about the organization and the position.

4. Answer applicant's questions about the organization and the position.

5. State that you both will benefit from using this plan.

6. Indicate you will be taking notes

MAKE TRANSITION TO KEY BACKGROUND REVIEW

Job and experience:_____Dates:_____

1. What were/are your main responsibilities and duties?

   Any changes in responsibilities?

2. How did you find and obtain this job?

3. Why did you (or why are you planning to) leave?

Appendix 5

FOCUSED INTERVIEWS
CRITICAL "MANAGER" QUESTIONS

Position: _____

Candidate: _____

Interview date: _____ With: _____

STAFF LEADERSHIP

1. Have you ever led task forces, committees, or groups that did not report to you but from whom you had to get work? What did you do to get what you wanted?

SITUATION	APPROACH	RESULT

2. What are some of the most difficult one-on-one meetings you have had with other members of your staff? Why were they difficult?

DIFFICULT MEETING(S)	HOW HANDLED	RESULT

CREATIVITY

1. What are some of the most imaginative or innovative things you have done in your present position?

SITUATION	ACTION	RESULT

2. What kinds of problems have people recently called on you to solve? Tell me about your contribution to solving the(se) problem(s).

PROBLEM	SOLUTION	RESULT

ATTENTION TO DETAIL

1. Describe your system for controlling errors in *your* work?

SYSTEM	ACTION	RESULT

2. We've all had times when we just couldn't get everything done on time. When and why has this happened to you?

SITUATION	ACTION	RESULT

JUDGMENT

1. Give me two examples of good decisions you have made in the past 6 months. What were the alternatives? Why were they good decisions?

SITUATION	DECISION (ALTERNATIVE)	RESULT

2. What were the toughest decisions you had to make while in your present position?

SITUATION	DECISION (ALTERNATIVE)	RESULT

ADAPTABILITY

1. Tell me about some situations in your job at _____
   where you had to abruptly change what you were doing. What did you do? How did it
   affect you?

SITUATION	REACTION	EFFECT

2. Which bosses have you worked most effectively for and why?

SITUATION	REACTION	EFFECT

3. Which bosses have been the hardest to work for?

SITUATION	REACTION	EFFECT

Finally, why are you the most qualified candidate for this position?

20 FACTOR TEST

Here are the 20 questions the Internal Revenue Service uses to determine whether workers are company employees or independent contractors. The IRS considers any "yes" answer to be evidence of an employer–employee relationship.

1. Do you provide the worker with instructions as to when, where, and how work is performed?
2. Did you train the worker to have the job performed correctly?
3. Are the worker's services a vital part of your company's operations?
4. Is the person prevented from delegating work to others?
5. Is the worker prohibited from hiring, supervising, and paying assistants?
6. Does the worker perform services for you on a regular and continuous basis?
7. Do you set the hours of service for the worker?
8. Does the person work full-time for your company?
9. Does the worker perform duties on your company's premises?
10. Do you control the order and sequence of the work performed?
11. Do you require workers to submit oral or written reports?
12. Do you pay the worker by the hour, week, or month?
13. Do you pay the worker's business and travel expenses?
14. Do you furnish tools or equipment for the worker?
15. Does the worker lack a "significant investment" in tools, equipment, and facilities?
16. Is the worker insulated from suffering a loss as a result of the activities performed for your company?
17. Does the worker perform services solely for your firm?
18. Does the worker not make services available to the general public?
19. Do you have the right to discharge the worker at will?
20. Can the worker end the relationship without incurring any liability?

Reprinted from Internal Revenue Service, "20 Factor Test."

Appendix 7

SAFETY AND MAINTENANCE CHECKLIST

GENERAL

Emergency procedures are posted in each room.
Signs are posted on proper use of equipment and rules of facility.
Floor is properly cleaned and maintained to prevent slips, trips, and falls.
Exercise class equipment is maintained for safety and easy access.

STRETCHING AREA

Safety

Weight benches and equipment areas are free of stray mats.
No large gaps are between mats in stretching areas.

Maintenance

Mats are free of rips and tears.
Area is swept and disinfected.

LOCKER ROOMS

Safety

No lockers are broken.
Floor in shower area is clean.
Floormats are in place on slippery surfaces.
Blow dryers are in good working order.

Maintenance

No lockers are broken.
Lockers are checked for day-use violations.
Work for maintenance staff is checked.
Soap, toilet paper, and paper towel supplies are checked.

Spa Areas

Sauna—temperature: 170° to 180° Fahrenheit; humidity: 5% relative
Steam room—temperature: 100° to 110° Fahrenheit; humidity: 100% relative
Whirlpool—temperature: 102° to 105° Fahrenheit

FREE WEIGHT AREA

Safety

Racks and weight standards are spaced properly to allow clear traffic flow.
Equipment is returned after use to avoid obstruction of pathway.
Safety equipment (belts, collars, safety bars) is available for use and stored properly.
Nonslip floor mats are in squat rack area.
Benches, weight racks, and standards are secured to the floor or wall.

Maintenance

Protective padding is free of rips, cracks, and tears.
Surfaces that contact human skin are properly cleaned and disinfected.
Securing bolts and apparatus parts (collars, curl bars, dumbbells) are tightened.
Olympic bars are lubricated and tightened to turn properly.
Nonfunctional apparatus and equipment are removed from area or locked out of service.

MACHINE AREA

Safety

Each workstation has easy access (minimum of 2 feet of space is required; 3 feet is optimum between machines).

Pins fit securely in weight stack.

Securing straps (seat belts) are functional.

There are no protruding screws or parts that need tightening or removal.

Maintenance

Area is free of loose bolts, screws, cables, and chains.

Parts and surfaces are properly lubricated and cleaned (guide rods on selected machines should be cleaned and lubricated two or three times a week).

Protective padding is free of rips, cracks, and tears.

Surfaces that contact human skin are properly cleaned and disinfected.

All parts are well lubricated and functioning smoothly.

Belts, chains, and cables are aligned with machine parts.

There are no worn parts (frayed cable, loose chains, worn bolts, or cracked joint screws).

CARDIOVASCULAR FITNESS AREA

Safety

Equipment is adequately spaced to allow free movement and traffic flow.

There are no protruding parts or screws that need tightening or removing.

Nonfunctional or broken equipment is removed or locked from use.

Maintenance

Surfaces that contact human skin are properly cleaned and disinfected.

All parts are well lubricated and functioning smoothly.

Machinery is clean.

Machinery is functioning properly.

All functions of equipment are in working order (e.g., batteries, dials; replaced when needed).

There are no frayed cables or belts.

From ACSM, Fitness facility inspection report. In *Health-Fitness facility standards and guidelines, 2nd ed.* (Champaign, IL: Human Kinetics).

Appendix 8

FITNESS FACILITY INSPECTION REPORT

Site: _____ Date: _____

Inspector: _____

S = Satisfactory   U = Unsatisfactory   NA = Not Applicable

	S	U	NA
STAFFING AND SUPERVISION			
1. Qualified personnel are present and supervising members on floor.			
2. Staff are dressed in proper uniform with name tags.			
3. Staff are available and accessible to members.			
4. Staff are versed on:			
(a) Evacuation procedures			
(b) Membership procedures and policies			
(c) Incident procedures			
STAFF TECHNICAL SKILLS			
5. Staff demonstrate ability to interpret health screening form.			
6. Staff are versed on site's policy for physician consent recommendation and requirement.			
7. Staff demonstrate ability to measure blood pressure accurately.			
8. Staff demonstrate ability to describe and measure skinfold site.			
9. Staff are able to describe procedures for all phases of sub-maximal VO$_2$ test.			
10. Demonstrate ability to provide equipment instruction.			
EXERCISE AREA APPEARANCE AND CLEANLINESS			
11. Exercise areas are clean and orderly.			
12. Equipment is adequately spaced and stored.			
13. Equipment is clean and in working order.			
14. Out-of-service equipment is labeled properly and removed from floor.			
15. Equipment manufacturer instructions are posted on equipment and in good condition.			
16. Electrical cords are properly secured.			
17. Equipment mats are clean.			
18. Mirrors and walls are clean and free of marks.			
19. Cleaning supplies are readily available and labeled appropriately.			
20. Magazines are stored in proper areas.			
LOCKER ROOM AREAS			
21. Wet areas are safe.			
22. Wet areas are sanitary.			
23. Lockers are clean (in/out) and doors are closed.			

229

	S	U	NA

24. Amenities are adequately stocked.
25. Carpet and matting are clean and properly secured.
26. Mirrors are clean and properly secured.
27. Sauna, whirlpool, and pool are set at correct temperature.
28. Sauna, whirlpool, and pool rules are posted.
29. Whirlpool and pool chemical readings are performed, recorded, and appropriate.
30. Paint, wallpaper, wall fixtures, and ceramic tiles are in good condition.

EMERGENCY PREPARATIONS

31. Emergency and evacuation procedures are posted in all appropriate locations.
32. Fire extinguishers are present with valid inspections.
33. Emergency lighting is tested and functional.

BULLETIN BOARDS AND SIGNS

34. Facility hours are posted.
35. Group exercise schedule is posted.
36. Facility staff biographies and pictures are posted.
37. All permanent signs are laminated.
38. Information is current, neat, free of mistakes, and health related.

OFFICE AREA

39. Area appears neat and orderly.
40. All operations, personnel, and other manuals are present.
41. Membership applications and information are available.

HEALTH PROMOTION INFORMATION

42. Health promotion information is available to members.
43. Past and present program evaluations and information are accessible.

RISK MANAGEMENT INFORMATION

44. Coding system for high-risk members is properly maintained.
45. Opening and closing procedures checklist is present and in use.
46. Equipment and facility maintenance and repairs are documented.
47. Building management notification is documented.
48. Emergency and first aid supplies are adequately stocked, available, and documented.
49. Staff CPR certifications are current and on file.
50. Staff first aid certifications are current and on file.
51. Additional required staff certifications are current and on file.

S	U	NA

52. Incident reports are properly documented and filed.

53. Staff training is performed and documented.

54. Emergency drills are performed quarterly and documented (one must be unannounced).

55. Emergency system is tested and documented.

56. OSHA materials checklist is complete.

57. Vendor insurance certificates are current and on file.

58. Professional services agreements are current and on file.

MEMBERSHIP DOCUMENTATION

59. Member files contain the following information with signatures: medical history, informed consent, waiver, and emergency contact.

60. Member records are locked.

61. Membership tracking systems are in place.

62. Manager is versed on procedures for accurate membership record keeping.

63. Fitness assessment paperwork is complete and accurate.

64. Staff comments and initials are on workout cards.

FINANCIAL DOCUMENTATION

65. Cash and valuables are properly secured.

66. Daily transactions are properly documented.

67. Petty cash and checkbook are balanced, with records and receipts present.

68. Wellness services deposit records are available.

69. Payroll deduction is reconciled.

70. Vendor accounts and billings are updated and organized.

COMMENTS:

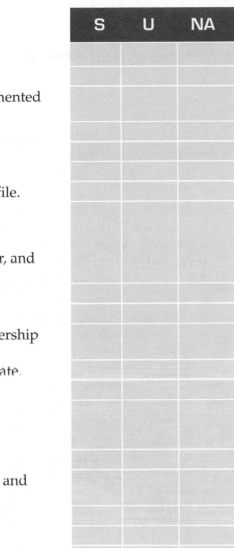

Appendix 9

BLOODBORNE PATHOGENS

Q: What are bloodborne pathogens and where are they found?

A: Bloodborne pathogens are microorganisms that are present in human blood and can cause disease in humans. These pathogens include, but are not limited to, hepatitis B (HBV) and human immunodeficiency virus (HIV).

These microorganisms are found in semen, vaginal secretion, any fluid visibly contaminated with blood, and all body fluids in situations where it is difficult or impossible to differentiate.

Q: How can they be contracted?

A: Bloodborne pathogens can cause infection by entering your body in a variety of ways, including open cuts, nicks, skin abrasions, dermatitis, acne, and the mucous membranes of your mouth, eyes, or nose.

Q: How can we be exposed at work?

A: You can become infected by accidentally injuring yourself with a sharp object that is contaminated. Sharp objects may be broken glass, sharp metal, needles, and knives. Bloodborne diseases can also be transmitted indirectly. Indirect transmission can happen when you touch an object or surface contaminated with blood or other materials and transfer the infection to your mouth, eyes, nose, or open skin.

Contaminated surfaces are a major cause of the spread of hepatitis. HBV can survive on environmental surfaces dried and at room temperatures for at least 1 week.

Q: How can we protect ourselves?

A: You can protect yourself from bloodborne pathogens by adopting the concept of universal precautions: Know where all personal protective equipment is kept and use them on all occasions of possible contact with contaminated substances. If an exposure incident occurs, get the HBV vaccination within 24 hours of exposure. Decontaminate all surfaces that have or possibly have been infected with bloodborne pathogens by using 10 to 1 (water to bleach) solution to remove the presence of contaminated microorganisms.

Q: What should we do if we have an "exposure incident"?

A: If you have been exposed to blood or body fluids you must do the following:

1. Use soap and water to wash the parts of your body that have been contaminated.

2. Report the incident to your supervisor. Early action can prevent the development of hepatitis B by obtaining the HBV vaccination and enable affected workers to track potential HIV infection.

3. Complete an incident report with details of the accident. Keep a copy in the site files and forward the original to your home office and human resource director.

Q: How do I decontaminate surfaces exposed to bloodborne pathogens?

A: If you are faced with cleaning up blood or body fluids, wear appropriate personal protective equipment, use a solution of one part bleach to two parts water, disinfect mops and cleaning tools after the job is done, and dispose of all contaminated protective equipment.

Source: Occupational Safety and Health Standards for General Industry (29 CFR PART 1910) dated Feb. 3, 1997.

Adapted from "Bloodborne Pathogens, What You Really Need to Know," YMCA of Metropolitan Washington, 112 16th St. NW, Suite 720, Washington, DC 20036.

DEFINITIONS

Bloodborne pathogens:

Pathogenic microorganisms that are present in human blood and can cause disease in humans. These pathogens include, but are not limited to, hepatitis B (HBV) and human immunodeficiency virus (HIV).

Contaminated:

The presence or reasonably anticipated presence of blood or other potentially infectious materials on an item or surface.

Decontamination:

The use of physical or chemical means to remove, inactivate, or destroy bloodborne pathogens on a surface or item to the point where they are no longer capable of transmitting infectious particles and the surface or item is rendered safe for handling, use, or disposal.

Exposure incident:

A specific eye, mouth, or mucous membrane, nonintact skin, or parenteral contact with blood or other potentially infectious materials that result from the performance of an employee's duties.

HIV and HBV:

Human immunodeficiency virus and hepatitis B virus.

Parenteral:

Piercing mucous membranes or the skin barrier through such events as needlesticks, human bites, cuts, and abrasions (an opening in the skin).

Personal protective equipment:

Specialized clothing or equipment worn by an employee for precaution against a hazard. These items include rubber gloves, eye goggles, and CPR protectors.

Universal precautions:

An approach to infection control. According to this concept, all human blood and certain human body fluids are treated as if known to be infectious for HIV, HBV, and other bloodborne pathogens.

Source: Occupational Safety and Health Standards for General Industry (29 CFR PART 1910) dated Feb. 3, 1997.

Appendix 10

INCIDENT REPORT

DATE

Month	Day	Year	Time of Incident	Facility name and location
			AM	
			PM	

MEMBER INFORMATION

First Name

Last Name

Agency/Division   Room Number

Office Phone #   Home Phone #

Age   M _____ F _____

Contacts made: (check all that apply)
Emergency medical system ___
Building security ___
Health unit ___
Name(s) of emergency responders:

Time of initial call:

Times of additional calls (if necessary):
1. _____ 2. _____ 3. _____

Time of EMS arrival:
Time of EMS departure:
Taken to hospital?   Yes ___   No ___

INCIDENT INFORMATION

Location of incident:

Bleeding injury: Yes ___   No ___

Description of injury:

Other visible injuries: Yes ___   No ___

Detailed description of incident and action taken by staff:

Member signature verifying incident details:

Date: Month   Day   Year

INCIDENT INFORMATION

Action taken to prevent in future:

WITNESS

Name of first witness

Agency/Division

Office Phone #   Home Phone #

Description of incident by witness:

Name of second witness

Agency/Division

Office Phone #   Home Phone #

Description of incident by witness:

Signature of witness:

Signature of witness:

Form submitted by: (print)   (Signature)   Date: Month   Day   Year

FOLLOW-UP

Follow-up performed by:

Date of follow-up: Month   Day   Year

Additional comments:

Appendix 11

POPULAR WEB SITES

American Cancer Society —www.cancer.org

American College of Sports Medicine—www.acsm.org

American Council on Exercise—www.acefitness.org

American Diabetes Association—www.diabetes.org

American Dietetic Association—www.eatright.org

American Heart Association—www.americanheart.org

American Journal of Health Promotion—www.healthpromotionjournal.com

American Medical Association—www.ama-assn.org

American Psychiatric Association—www.psych.org

Centers for Disease Control and Prevention—www.cdc.gov

Center for Nutrition Policy and Promotion—www.usda.gov/cnpp/

Fitness Management—www.fitnessmanagement.com

Human Kinetics—www.HumanKinetics.com

IDEA—www.ideafit.com

InteliHealth—www.intelihealth.com

International Health, Racquet & Sportsclub Association—www.ihrsa.org

Mayo Clinic Health Oasis—www.mayo.edu

National Agricultural Library—Food and Nutrition Information—www.nal.usda.gov/fnic

National Health Information Center—www.health.gov/nhic

National Institutes of Health—www.nih.gov

National Wellness Institute, Inc.—www.nationalwellness.org

The Physician and Sportsmedicine Online—www.physsportsmed.com

Reuters Health Information Services—www.reutershealth.com

Tufts University Nutrition Navigator—www.navigator.tufts.edu

United States National Library of Medicine—www.nlm.nih.gov

Wellness Councils of America—www.welcoa.org

World Health Organization—www.who.int

Appendix 12

SELF-EVALUATION/LEADERSHIP DEVELOPMENT

Name: _____ Date: _____

You are asked to fill out this form completely and bring it to our next meeting. During the meeting, we will discuss whether you are ready to continue to the next stage of management and the reasons for this decision. Comparison of your evaluation of yourself with my evaluation of you will assist in an overall assessment and help to set the foundation for your next level of development.

What are your main strengths? _____

_____

What things do you think you need to improve to increase your potential for growth? _____

_____

_____

Please give careful consideration to how well the following characteristics apply to you?

1 = Not at all   2 = Slightly well   3 = Moderately well

4 = Rather well   5 = Extremely well

	1	2	3	4	5
Considered as a loyal manager					
Treats others with respect and consideration					
Uses diplomacy and tact when dealing with others					
Is able to deal effectively with difficult issues					
Has the respect of coworkers					
Is a team player					
Lends assistance to others in the group on a regular basis					
Cooperates with others					
Is a leader among peers					
Has a positive influence on the morale of the group					
Tries to resolve conflicts or complaints					
Accepts change with an open mind					
Accepts responsibility for mistakes					
Handles stressful situations well					
Follows through on commitments					
Is able to organize tasks for maximum efficiency					
Is able to work well with minimal supervision					
Displays interest in improving work habits					
Makes thoughtful suggestions that lead to improvement					
Thinks problems through clearly					
Seeks answers to questions					
Has good verbal communication skills					
Has good written communication skills					

	1	2	3	4	5

Attendance has always been good

Sets an example by returning promptly from breaks and lunch

Sets an example by following set policies and procedures

Is attentive to details

Can be trusted in all avenues of managerial operations

Is seen as one who sets a positive example continuously

Has the training that you have received so far in this position helped you? If so, how has it helped? If not, how could it be improved? _____

_____

_____

_____

After carefully reviewing the ratings that you have given yourself on this form, do you believe you are ready to progress to another level if available? Why? _____

_____

_____

_____

Employee: _____

Manager: _____

Dated: _____

Appendix 13

KEY MANAGEMENT PRACTICES IN FORTUNE 100 BEST COMPANIES

RECRUITMENT, SELECTION, AND RETENTION

Telecommuting full-time or 1 or more days per week

Nontraditional career tracks

Four-day work weeks—three 12-hour days and every other Sunday

No layoff policy (18 companies)

Rigorous screening for core ideology and "tightness of fit"

PARTICIPATION

Employees can make a direct connection between their work and the company's mission

Employee councils take up complaints

Core ideology is institutionalized: seminar focus and content translated into employee reviews and promotions

Give managers the authority and freedom to run their departments as if it was their own business

Social activities that reinforce corporate philosophy and team

Emphasize individual effort within the context of the collective effort

RECOGNITION

Using employee ideas to solve problems

Ensure employees believe their opinions count (annual Chairman's Award: $5,000 in cash and $2,500 in travel expenses)

Respect and concern for individual employees is a core ideology

Recognize individual initiative and innovation

Internal or external customer feedback loops

Service orientation reinforced by tangible rewards and penalties

Cash awards or public recognition for cost savings and service enhancements that can be re-produced in other business units

Profiling employees who tried something that worked really well

Tips and ideas generated by employees published in internal magazine

Productivity recognition with special privileges and designation

LEARNING AND GROWING

5% of work time spent in training

Extensive training programs (best in industry)

Strong commitment to education (100 hours per year for manager and 2+ hours per year for employee)

Program for employees to try out new jobs in the company

Tuition aid up to $9,600 per year

Researchers allotted 15% of their time to pursue any project that interests them

EXCITING WORK

Employees given the opportunity to do what they do best every day

Culture that promotes fun and closer work relationships with colleagues

Easy-going work environment

Organization is willing to change everything about itself except its basic philosophy to adapt and move forward

Urges continual change (new directions, new methods, new strategies)

Created fierce competitions between product lines to stimulate progress

Created internal venture capital fund

CUTTING-EDGE TECHNOLOGY

State-of-the-art information systems infrastructure

Satellite communications to spread information around company as soon as possible

Invented new technology processes and invested in the most advanced technologies

ADVANCEMENT

Chance to change careers within same company

Extremely strong commitments to promotion from within

Provide employees with long-range career opportunities and suitable projects on which to work

WORK/LIFE

Ability to balance work and family obligations through flexible schedules

On-site child care

Child care subsidies

Child care resource and referral services

Backup child care center

Sick child day care

Elder care resource and referral services

Nursing home care insurance (spouses, parents, grandparents)

24-hour work/family hotline

Reimbursement for travel-related child care

COMPENSATION

Substantial employee referral bonuses ($1,500–$10,000)

Good profit sharing. Distributions made each quarter (multiple companies)

Paid time for volunteer activities

$10,000 "Lifecycle" account (first house, first baby, college tuition)

75% match, or approximately 6% on 401K

100% match, or approximately 8% of pay

ESOPs

HEALTH BENEFITS

Employer pays entire health insurance premium (multiple companies)

Domestic partner benefits

Free annual physical

$50 to take physical; $200 for healthy results

12 weeks paid maternity leave

10K adoption aid

Postpartum RN sent to home for 3 days after delivery

VACATION BENEFITS

Extra vacation at 10 years service and every 5 years thereafter (10 to 35 days)

1 week paid leave for new dads and adoptive parents

6 months family leave for new mothers or adoptive parents

Unlimited time off to care for sick child

Up to 48 hours per year to use for emergencies with the kids

13 paid holidays per year

WOMEN AND MINORITIES

Women hold > 50% of the top jobs

Active caucuses of women, African Americans, Hispanics, gays, and lesbians

Strong support network for women managers

CONVENIENCE SERVICES

Free beverages and food at all times

Concierge

General store

Film processing

Dry cleaning

Travel agent

Auto repair

Van pool or public transportation subsidies

Bank or ATM

Athletic facilities or fitness and wellness centers (extended hours, intramural leagues, on-site exercise classes)

Masseur or certified massage therapy

SOCIAL ACTIVITIES

Companywide events

Holiday party for employees' children

Annual teamwork day

Company golf outing

OTHER

Full-time benefits for part-time employees

No time clocks

Company support to employees with personal crises

Appendix 14

SAMPLE HEART CHECK QUESTIONS:
SMOKING-CESSATION PROGRAMS

Does/did the worksite provide smoking-cessation programs and services during the previous 24 months? If yes, continue. Does/did the worksite do any of the following:

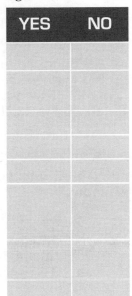

	YES	NO
Provide or subsidize the use of the nicotine patch or other nicotine substitute projects?		
Conduct the program on an annual basis (at least once during the previous 12 months)?		
Subsidize the program by at least 50%?		
Provide the program both on-site and off-site?		
Use credentialed instructors?		
Use more than one form of program delivery (e.g., self-study materials such as computers, video- or audiocassettes, or self-paced learning manuals)?		
Promote the availability of programs through at least two regular communication channels (e.g., newsletter or bulletin boards)?		
Provide program access during company paid time (not lunchtime)?		

Appendix 15

EXAMPLE OF A FINAL REPORT COMMUNICATION SECTION

MULTIPLE TOOLS AND PATHWAYS
Recommendations

Need to continue to meet with the communication specialists of the workforce effectiveness department to ensure that your current communication tools fold into their look and quality. Make sure that you are using these new resources to the maximum and that the health and wellness message is throughout their efforts.

A written communication strategy needs to be developed that systematically promotes and markets the headquarters program. This strategy should continue to utilize the newsletter, administration bulletins, easels, and program flyers. Components of this strategy would be

Clear description of each communication vehicle and its development and distribution processes, and who it is intended to reach (e.g., employee, management)

A timeline that guides the development and distribution of all components within the strategy

Evaluation tools developed and described to ensure highest quality and maximum exposure

Specific methods that will be used to report the programs progress to management (see evaluation section)

NEWSLETTER
Recommendations

You might consider buying newsletter software or meeting with a computer specialist who could help you evaluate the newsletter potential of your word-processing software. There might be an employee volunteer who could help you write and format your newsletter. The newsletter should continue to be published and distributed to employees six times a year.

You and the employees need to solve the distribution problems experienced with the newsletter. Try several solutions to arrive at the best one.

The newsletter should continue to raise awareness, increase knowledge, teach skills, motivate change, reinforce behaviors, support behaviors, and promote upcoming programs. The annual evaluation of the newsletter will allow you to measure how it is doing. A random evaluation annually on 3% of the population will give you a good idea of the effectiveness of the newsletter.

The mission of the program should be apparent in every newsletter, and several times during the year a review of the annual goals should be given to ensure that employees and managers understand why the program is important.

You should also consider putting a quarterly program schedule in appropriate newsletters. This schedule will provide employees with information about upcoming programs and give them an opportunity to plan their schedule so that they can participate.

Consider mailing the newsletter interoffice, with notes attached, to managers you are trying to influence on certain projects.

Periodically review external newsletters for potential use and benchmarking.

NEW EMPLOYEE ORIENTATION

Recommendations

You need to sit through a new employee orientation and review the current process first-hand. Such participation will give you some ideas on how and what the health and wellness component needs to look like.

Try different promotional pieces about the program to ensure they work before having them put into a book or brochure. You might consider a video that not only talks about the different aspects of the program but also lets different levels of employees talk about what health and wellness means to them. A video cannot be longer than 7 to 12 minutes. It might be a video sent to new employees that they can view with their families.

During the orientation process the new employees should be given the mission and goals of the program.

Consider having volunteers call all new employees to welcome them to the program.

Field employee orientations to the program would depend on the extent that the program was implemented at a location. If you base these orientations on the headquarters orientation process, it will help tie the remote and headquarters programs together and focus them on the overall mission and program goals.

Index

Note: The italicized *f* and *t* following page numbers refer to figures and tables, respectively.

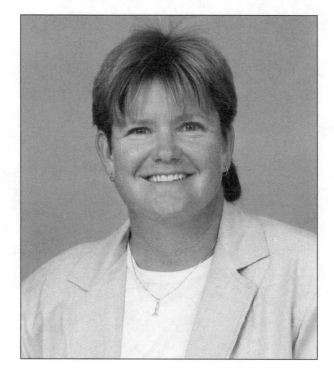

Carolyn C. Cox, PhD, CHES, is an associate professor of health science at Truman State University in Kirksville, Missouri. She is respected in the field of worksite health promotion and frequently serves as a reviewer for textbook publishers on the topic.

Extensively published and well practiced as a presenter of research on worksite health promotion, Cox is a member of the American College of Sports Medicine's Alliance of Health Fitness Professionals, chair of the Missouri Governor's Council on Physical Fitness and Health's Worksite Health Promotion Task Force, and a fellow of the former Association for Worksite Health Promotion.

Dr. Cox also is an active member of the National Wellness Institute and the American Alliance for Health Education of the American Alliance for Health, Physical Education, Recreation and Dance (AAHPERD). The Central District and Missouri Chapter of AAHPERD named her the College/University Health Education Professional of the Year for 2002. Dr. Cox enjoys fitness walking, strength training, and cycling in her free time.